*HOW MYTHS
ABOUT WEIGHT LOSS
ARE KEEPING US FAT —
AND THE TRUTH ABOUT
WHAT REALLY WORKS*

Supersized
LIES

ROBERT J. DAVIS, PhD

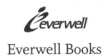

Everwell Books

Published by Everwell Books, an imprint of MediVista Media, LLC
www.everwell.com

View all the author's titles at healthyskeptic.com.

Cover design by Michael Rehder / rehderandcompanie.com
Interior design by Alex Head / thedraftlab.com

ISBN: 978-1-7369677-0-6
ePub ISBN: 978-1-7369677-1-3
Library of Congress Control Number: 2021906457

Printed in the United States of America

For Daniel,
who's winning the battle

CONTENTS

INTRODUCTION

Horace Fletcher was a rich man, but there was one thing he couldn't buy: life insurance. Standing 5 feet, 7 inches and weighing over 200 pounds, he was deemed too fat to be insurable. After applying and getting rejected several times, the bon vivant businessman came up with a way to slim down that would put him in the annals of weight-loss history.

Fletcher's method involved chewing. And chewing—and chewing. In fact, he chewed every mouthful of food until it completely liquefied and lost its flavor. Some foods had to be munched more than 700 times before reaching oblivion. After four months of this interminable routine, Fletcher had dropped more than 40 pounds and lost 7 inches off his waist.

Had he lived today, Fletcher might have become a YouTube sensation. But the year was 1898, so he spread the word about the benefits of ceaseless chomping by writing, lecturing, and giving press interviews. Having been sick and sluggish at his previous weight, the former athlete publicly displayed his chewing-induced vigor with stunts like backward flips off a diving board, lifting a man on his shoulders, and cycling 190 miles.

Thanks to Fletcher's showmanship and charisma, his chewing regimen went viral in early 20th-century America and Europe. Luminaries such as John D. Rockefeller, Thomas Edison, and Henry Ford embraced the practice—dubbed "Fletcherism"—as did Dr. John Harvey Kellogg, the nation's most famous physician. People formed chewing clubs and held parties to "Fletcherize." (What was a noon-time chewing party called? A muncheon!) As Susan Yager writes in her book *The Hundred Year Diet*, "Sing Sing prison inmates, schoolchildren, the highest of high society, and the middle-most of the middle class all chewed and chewed."

The Fletcherism craze died when its inventor did in 1919, but it lives on today as an example of a silly and unsound way to lose weight that nevertheless gained wide acceptance. Certainly it's not the only one. History is filled with laughable weight-loss "cures"—everything from bath salts and soaps that could supposedly wash away fat to cigarettes ("Reach for a Lucky instead of a sweet," said ads for Lucky Strike cigarettes in the 1920s) to tapeworm eggs, which people ingested to consume the food in their intestines.

Today, we're far more sophisticated about weight control than our forebears who fell for such hokum. Or so we think. In reality, much of the conventional wisdom about weight and obesity from experts and the media—and what many of us accept as established fact—is unproven or flat-out wrong.

No one has been more outspoken on this issue than David Allison, an iconoclastic obesity researcher who's dean of the Indiana University School of Public Health–Bloomington. A groundbreaking paper he coauthored in the *New England Journal of Medicine* identified a number of widely believed obesity-related myths and unproven assumptions, which the study concluded are "pervasive in both scientific literature and the popular press."

While Allison says scientific knowledge regarding obesity has increased and that there have been advances in the field, he thinks that much of what we hear is "nonsense and conjecture that masquerades as fact."

Whether it's intermittent fasting or low-carb diets, fat-burning foods or weight-loss supplements, many of today's "scientific" approaches are actually no more substantiated than Fletcherism for achieving long-term weight control. While they may help us lose weight for a few months or even a year, they almost always fail eventually. In some cases, they actually make matters worse and, like cigarettes and tapeworm eggs, can cause other harms.

These misguided ideas and practices—what they are, where they came from, and how they're hindering our quest to lose weight—are what this book is about.

Sad Stats

According to government surveys, the percentage of Americans trying to lose weight is on the rise, and roughly half of respondents say they've attempted to slim down in the past year. Three-quarters report that they've tried to lose weight at some point in their lives.

We're spending big bucks to do so. By the latest estimates, the weight-loss industry—which includes diet foods and drinks, commercial weight-loss plans, health clubs, diet books, drugs and supplements, bariatric surgery, and medically supervised programs—is now worth more than $60 billion in the United States.

As that figure has continued to balloon over the past several decades, so have our waistlines. According to the most recent data, more than 42 percent of US adults now have obesity, up from 30 percent in 2000. During that time, the rate of people with severe obesity has nearly doubled, reaching almost 10 percent.

Here are more sobering statistics to chew on:

- ➲ In 1990, no state had an obesity rate over 20 percent. Today, all 50 do, including those with the nation's "leanest" populations, such as Colorado and Hawaii.

- ➲ In 1980, the obesity rate among children and adolescents was 5.5 percent. By 2000, it had risen to 14 percent. Today it stands at 19 percent.

- ➲ More than 70 percent of American adults are now classified as either overweight or obese.

- ➲ Worldwide, about 2 billion adults are overweight or obese.

As if those figures weren't depressing enough, consider the high failure rates for long-term weight loss. Studies show that dieters gain back more than half of lost weight, on average, within two years and 80 percent of it within five years. Overall, 97 percent of people eventually regain at least some of the weight they've lost. As the joke goes, "I try to lose weight, but it keeps finding me!"

By whatever measure you choose, our efforts to control our weight are a colossal failure.

You would think that this fiasco would lead to some kind of reckoning and a reevaluation of what we're doing. Instead, many obesity experts, weight-loss gurus, and others who dispense advice just keep pushing the same failed solutions.

For example, in a study noting the paradox that more people are continuing to get heavier while attempting to lose weight, the researchers don't question the effectiveness of measures like eating less and exercising more. Instead they blame us, concluding that many people "might not have actually implemented weight loss strategies or [have] applied a minimal level of effort." In other words, the problem is that we're not trying hard enough.

Such an attitude is reminiscent of responses to medical treatment failures in bygone eras. When ineffective measures like bloodletting and mercury didn't work, doctors didn't blame the treatments. Instead, they often doubled down and administered the gruesome remedies even more aggressively. Just as hapless patients did back then, we frequently go along with experts' appeals to stay the course when it comes to our weight.

You're Biased!

So if there's no solid evidence for many weight-control remedies, and we can see that they're not working, why do so many people, including researchers, health experts, and the general public, continue to cling to them?

David Allison says one reason is cognitive biases, which are systematic errors in how we think. All people—even the smartest scientists—exhibit these biases, usually without realizing it. They include:

- ➲ **Mere exposure effect.** When people are repeatedly exposed to an idea, they're more likely to believe it. So if we hear over and over, for example, that weight control boils down to eating less and exercising more, we tend to accept it as true. The same goes for experts who encounter beliefs that are repeated in scientific papers and forums.

- ➲ **Bandwagon effect.** Also known as groupthink, this bias makes us more likely to adopt ideas or practices because everyone else seems to be on board. If the prevailing wisdom appears to be that, say, carbs are the main cause of weight gain, people tend to follow the herd and embrace the belief.

⊃ **Allegiance effect.** This entails a strong attachment to a particular approach—whether keto, paleo, gluten-free, or something else—and a belief that it's superior to all others. When consumers or experts closely identify with a particular camp, they tend to dig in and have a hard time letting go. If confronted with evidence that refutes their belief, they may ignore it and instead embrace only information that supports their position—a phenomenon known as *confirmation bias*.

⊃ **Reasonableness bias.** When something sounds reasonable, we have a greater tendency to believe it's true. For example, eating breakfast seems like a sensible thing to do, so people are more likely to accept it as a valid weight-loss strategy without questioning it.

⊃ **Wishful thinking.** When we badly want something to succeed and it doesn't, we may continue to believe that it will eventually work, despite a lack of evidence to support our belief. Wishful thinking prompts experts to stick to the same strategies, and consumers to try diets over and over. For both, the hope is that doing the same things will somehow lead to a different result, which, as the old saying goes, is the definition of insanity.

Social media often reinforces these biases by increasing our exposure to particular ideas and giving the false impression that "everyone" agrees, when in fact there may be agreement only among the relatively small subset of people whose posts social media algorithms put in front of us.

This selective exposure to information can also create and harden allegiances to weight-loss creeds by surrounding us virtually with like-minded people. If you're inclined to believe, say, that veganism is the answer to weight control, you're likely to end up in a vegan echo chamber that further bolsters your belief.

In addition, hearing about other people's weight-loss triumphs through social media can lead us to falsely conclude that a particular approach will succeed for us because it worked (or seemed to) for them.

When those other people are celebrities, the effect can be especially powerful. Many of us form so-called parasocial relationships with famous people, which are basically one-way friendships. Following them on Twitter and hearing about their every move, we may feel that we know them and can trust them as credible sources of information. Plus, we see their slim, beautiful bodies as evidence that they know what they're talking about, even though in reality, celebrities' weight-related practices and pronouncements are often scientifically baseless.

The news media, which are a leading source of information about weight control for many of us, may also feed certain biases and mislead us, especially through coverage of research. Too often, news reports overstate the importance and definitiveness of studies, drawing sweeping conclusions that aren't justified while giving short shrift to key limitations.

One such limitation is the type of research. Not all studies are created equal. There's a hierarchy, with test-tube and animal research yielding the least definitive evidence. When reporting such studies, news stories may give a false impression with statements like "a new study says green tea

7

helps you lose weight," which fails to make it clear that the "you" in the study were obese mice and the findings may not apply to people.

Likewise, news stories often use misleading language when referring to observational studies, which show associations between two things—say, exercise and lower weight. If, based on such an association, a report tells us exercise *causes* weight loss, that's deceptive because observational studies can't prove cause and effect. It could be that exercisers have other habits, like eating a healthy diet, that are actually responsible for their lower weight. While researchers try to control for such factors, their methods aren't foolproof.

Randomized trials, which assign participants to receive either a treatment (such as a particular diet) or a placebo, are considered the gold standard of studies because they're able to prove causality. Still, they too can have shortcomings that limit their believability or relevance. For example, a trial that lasts four weeks can't tell us whether an intervention leads to long-term weight loss, and a study in which all the subjects are college students may not apply to middle-aged and older people. Often media reports give little or no attention to crucial details such as these.

Journalists can fall short when covering research for a number of reasons, including a lack of scientific training, tight deadlines, limited space (or time in broadcasting), and the need to make bold statements—in other words, to sensationalize—to grab the audience's attention.

As a journalist, I certainly don't defend shoddy coverage and routinely point out examples in speeches to colleagues. But to be fair, the blame doesn't lie solely with journalists. Distorted press releases also play a role. In many cases, reporters take their cues from materials put out by universities and scientific journals, and research shows that these releases often contain the same types of exaggerations and omissions that we see in media coverage.

If you go back farther in the chain, you'll sometimes find that the studies themselves suffer from the same problems, with researchers' biases prompting them to overstate their findings or interpret the data in ways that are misleading. When these researchers are quoted in press releases or media reports, their spin typically goes unchallenged, giving us a skewed impression of reality.

It's not just cognitive biases that can lead to these kinds of misrepresentations by researchers. So can financial biases. Funding of weight-related studies by food companies, diet plans, pharmaceutical manufacturers, supplement makers, and others helps researchers survive professionally and allows them to conduct research that might not otherwise be possible. So it's easy to see why they would want to please their sponsors, or at least not bite the hand that feeds them.

Researchers typically insist that funding doesn't influence their work, and it's true that corporate sponsorship doesn't necessarily render a study invalid. But there is evidence that nutrition studies sponsored by the food industry more often report results favorable to funders' interests than studies without industry funding.

This may happen because researchers design their experiments in a way that's more likely to show benefits. They may frame the data to make those benefits appear as large or impressive as possible. Or they may emphasize findings that support the sponsor's interest and downplay or ignore those that don't. These nuances can be hard to detect and may not even be evident to the researchers themselves.

Of course, the effects of money extend far beyond researchers. As I mentioned earlier, weight loss is a multibillion-dollar business, and many players in the industry help perpetuate myths because doing so is in their financial interest. If commercial weight-loss companies and diet book authors can keep us believing there's a "best" diet, or food companies and supplement makers can keep alive the notion that the "right" products will magically melt away pounds, these sellers can keep taking our money. Because what they're selling usually doesn't work long term, the need for it never goes away. Nor do sellers' profits.

Truth or Consequences

One obvious consequence of weight-loss myths and misconceptions is wasted money and effort that could be spent on more effective strategies. This wouldn't be such an urgent problem if obesity were just a cosmetic issue. But in fact it's a matter of life and death.

The failure to control our weight is fueling a host of serious health problems, including an epidemic of type 2 diabetes. In addition, obesity is associated with an increased risk of heart disease, stroke, high blood pressure, osteoarthritis, sleep apnea, dementia, depression, fatty liver disease, gallbladder diseases, kidney disease, reproductive problems, certain cancers, and premature death. What's more, people with obesity are more prone to severe illness from the flu and COVID-19.

It's not just the upper extremes of weight that can give rise to health issues. In some research, gaining as little as 10 pounds between early and middle adulthood is linked to an increased risk of diabetes, cardiovascular disease, severe arthritis, and certain cancers, as well as decreased odds of healthy aging. Other research has found that putting on 20 or more pounds is associated with an elevated risk of premature death, especially as people hit their mid-50s and beyond.

Misguided approaches to weight control not only fail to adequately head off these threats but also pose their own risks. As I detail in this book, these can include increased cravings, decreased enjoyment of meals, disordered eating, weight cycling, stress, and liver damage, to name just a few.

Perhaps the most common side effect is weight stigma. Obesity myths contribute to it by reinforcing the false notion that we can control weight entirely through measures like strict dieting and exercise, and that people who don't succeed must be lazy, gluttonous, or lacking in self-discipline.

Reflecting this view, 75 percent of respondents in one survey named insufficient willpower as a barrier to weight loss, putting it ahead of all other contributors, including genetics. Similarly, readers responded to a *New York Times* column about rising obesity rates with comments such as these:

> "Simple solution: eat less, work out more. This is self-created, self-imposed. Absolutely no one to blame but the individual."

> "The fat/obese simply have no self control, discipline, or will to lead a healthy life. I've no sympathy for them as they have no respect for themselves."

> "What happened to self discipline? . . . Don't blame your poor choices on anything other than you."

Such attitudes are also common among health-care professionals. Acknowledging this reality, Dr. David Prologo of Emory University has penned an open apology to overweight patients told to lose weight with diet and exercise. "We have set them up to take the fall for our failed treatment approaches," he writes. "When they came to us with the truth about tolerability, we loudly discredited them and said they were mentally weak, noncompliant, or lazy."

While weight stigma undoubtedly has a pernicious effect on how society views and treats overweight people, it also negatively influences how they judge themselves. This internalized bias, which results in feelings of guilt, shame, and self-blame, can be especially harmful. Among other things, it's associated with depression, anxiety, low self-esteem, and binge eating, as well as a decreased likelihood of engaging in healthy behaviors like exercise. In such a way, internalized stigma not only damages people's health and quality of life but also makes weight control even more difficult.

That's what Angela experienced. After gaining 30 pounds in college, she was able to lose most of it. But maintaining the weight loss proved to be more difficult, in part because of an unhealthy relationship and a job that required a five-hour commute several times a week. Eventually Angela gained back all the weight, plus 30 pounds.

She quit the job, ended the relationship, ate less, and exercised. Though she was trying to do all the "right" things, she had trouble unloading all the extra weight. Angela blamed herself and felt anger toward her body for not responding to the measures that had worked before. "It caused me to hate my body," she says. The self-blame and anger led her to think "Why bother trying?" and to punish herself by overeating. Her self-esteem plummeted, worsening her underlying depression. "Seeing myself in the mirror," she says, "I had a lot of negative talk-back," which included "feeling like a failure and feeling ashamed of myself."

Her therapist challenged Angela to show the same compassion for herself that she showed to others. As part of this effort, Angela would ask herself, "What has my body given me today?" in order to shift the focus from what her body *prevented* her from doing to what it *helped* her do.

Today Angela tries to combat feelings of shame, anger, and failure by not worrying about hitting a certain number on the scale or fitting into a certain size. Instead, she focuses on what she can control and what she can do, like run, hike, and dance, and how she feels when she's doing it. In addition, she keeps a journal, which allows her to put her feelings into words and let go of some of the negative thoughts about herself and her weight.

All of this has helped put Angela on a healthier path physically and emotionally. In addition to walking regularly and eating a healthy diet that includes lots of vegetables, she now has greater insight into her own emotions and what's behind them—knowledge that, at age 30, has better equipped her to deal with not just her weight but other challenges in her life as well.

The Road Ahead

Throughout this book you'll see stories of real people like Angela who, in their battles to manage their weight, fell victim to the effects of misguided ideas but have found ways to overcome them. Unlike typical weight-related "successes" that we often read about, the victories of these folks lie not in how many pounds or inches they've lost, but in how they've gained awareness of the futility of conventional thinking and have forged other paths that are more effective for them.

Some experts say that instead of trying to change individuals' behavior, the focus should be on changing societal forces that contribute to obesity, such as gigantic restaurant portions, the availability of unhealthy, fattening foods everywhere we turn, and relentless marketing to prompt us to purchase them.

Unquestionably, factors like these play a significant role, and in this book I scrutinize some of the measures intended to address them, such as taxing soda purchases and requiring calorie counts on menus. But my main emphasis is on advice aimed at us personally. That's because while individual responsibility isn't the whole story regarding our weight, it's nevertheless a key part of it.

To deny this, as some do, implies that we're helpless victims incapable of exerting any personal control over our weight and health. That's simply not true. With the right strategies and the right expectations, we can in fact make meaningful and lasting changes in our own lives.

This empowerment begins with knowing what advice to heed and what to ignore. To that end, chapters 1 through 7 deal with myths and misconceptions related to restrictive diets, calorie counting, exercise, fat-burning foods, meal timing, supplements and pills, and ideal weight. In each case, I delve into the history of the advice, showing in some instances how ostensibly cutting-edge trends are actually retreads of old ideas.

In addition, drawing on my academic training in public health and epidemiology, I dissect the science, pointing out where and how specific claims deviate from the evidence. (I've documented everything with several hundred citations, so if you're inclined to check out the science for yourself or see how I reached my conclusions, have at it!) I also explain how unsupported claims undermine our weight-control efforts and, in some cases, lead to harm.

But this book isn't just about what's misleading or false. I also discuss what actually works, concluding each chapter with steps you can take to avoid wasting time, money, and effort. In the final chapter, I provide a comprehensive overview of effective strategies, which as you'll see are far less complicated than many of the "solutions" we often hear about. Still, you won't find a 30-day or 7-step weight-loss plan here because there's no such thing as a one-size-fits-all solution. Instead, I present a set of science-backed principles, which I hope can help you make more informed choices about the best ways to reach your own goals.

In "Myth or Truth?" sidebars along the way, you'll get quick takes on the veracity of statements that we frequently hear, such as: Some foods have "negative" calories; drinking lots of water promotes weight loss; fruit is fattening; high-sweat workouts burn more calories; and snacking is bad.

I should note that my focus throughout the book is adults. This is in no way meant to downplay or ignore childhood obesity and the importance of addressing it. But young people often require different approaches than adults, especially to promote a positive body image and prevent a lifetime of internalized weight stigma. Trying to squeeze all this into the book wouldn't do the material justice, so I leave it to others to address the topic.

...

One of my favorite cartoons, which appeared in the *New Yorker*, shows a woman in a bookstore walking by a section labeled "Diet Books." She sees that the shelves are divided into two sections—"Fiction" and "Nonfiction."

The cartoon, which gets a knowing laugh when I show it to audiences, captures the feelings that most of us have about not just diet books but weight-loss advice in general. My hope is that this book will help you separate fiction from nonfiction as you navigate your weight-loss journey, and set you on a path to success.

Chapter 1

PICK YOUR VILLAIN

*H*usky. *Full-seated. Spare tire.* They're words I vividly remember clothing store clerks and family friends using to describe my physique when I was a child. Though intended to be polite, the observations still stung because even at age 8, I knew exactly what they meant: I was fat.

In an effort to help me slim down, my mother instructed me to forgo bread. The advice reflected what she'd learned growing up, that starchy foods are the main culprit when it comes to weight. I complied with her directive (at least in her presence) even at my favorite restaurant and reluctantly removed the buns from my McDonald's hamburgers.

When I got to college in the 1980s and became interested in nutrition, I laughed as I recalled Mom's weight-loss prescription. According to what I was now learning, she'd had it backwards. The main cause of weight gain was fat, not starches. So she should have told me to skip the burger, not the bun.

Had I been an overweight child today, my mother—who keeps up with the latest nutrition thinking—might well have fingered a different culprit and put the kibosh instead on the sugary soda that I typically ordered with my hamburgers.

Luckily for me, I became thinner as I grew. But our society has not outgrown our insatiable desire to find a dietary villain that we can blame for our expanding waistlines. We lurch from one to another, from fat to carbs to gluten to soda. Or, depending on which diet you follow, the enemy might be animal products, legumes, cooked foods, acidic foods, or foods that our ancestors didn't eat.

It's human nature to gravitate toward good-versus-evil explanations for complex problems. We see the same phenomenon in other areas of life, including politics. While having a clearly defined enemy may satisfy our primal need for a simple narrative to make sense of things, it can do harm if it distracts us from what really matters.

That's what's happened in our battle with weight. We've been led down one dead end after another chasing elusive bad guys that keep changing. A variety of forces have cheered us on in this chase, including diet peddlers, the news media, and food manufacturers that are more than delighted to sell us all the fat-free, carb-free, or other enemy-free foods we can eat.

Nutrition researchers, obesity experts, and government agencies also bear responsibility for leading us astray by overstating the certainty of the science when it comes to culprits. What research does show is that weight-loss diets that demonize whole categories of foods may work in the short term, but in the long run, they're rarely sustainable. And they can make matters worse. As Dr. Yoni Freedhoff, author of *The Diet Fix*, puts it: "The notion that there's one causal food, or category of food, that is leading society to gain weight is a dangerous one."

Fat Phobia

The concept of off-limits foods has been around since the beginning of recorded history. After all, in the Bible it was forbidden fruit that led to the suffering of Adam and Eve and, according to the story, all of humanity. But few edible bogeymen have engendered such widespread fear and loathing as dietary fat.

The case against fat began in the 1950s, when scientist Ancel Keys launched the landmark Seven Countries Study and found that nations with higher intakes of saturated fat had higher rates of heart disease. Though anti-carb crusaders have posthumously accused Keys of rigging his research to prove what he wanted—as I said earlier, every narrative needs a villain—a white paper reviewing the facts reveals that charge to be false.

Keys' research along with other studies prompted a landmark report in 1977 by the US Senate Select Committee on Nutrition and Health Needs, which urged Americans to eat less fat and more complex carbohydrates. Named the "McGovern Report" after the committee's chairman, Senator George McGovern, it put a giant bull's-eye on the backs of high-fat foods like beef, eggs, whole milk, cheese, nuts, and butter.

While the focus was mainly on preventing heart disease, proponents of a low-fat diet pushed it as a way to control weight as well. The rationale was that, per gram, fat has more than twice as many calories as carbohydrates or protein. Also, the body converts excess dietary fat into stored fat relatively easily and uses less energy to process fat than carbs or protein, which means we absorb more of the calories from fat.

Support also came from studies in animals showing that when fed high-fat diets, they gain body fat and become obese. But the evidence for this in people was inconclusive. Nevertheless, the message fed to the public was unambiguous: Eating fat makes you fat. Promoted by nutritionists, news reports, and diet books, the mantra became a familiar refrain of the 1980s and '90s.

Among those leading the charge against fat has been Dr. Dean Ornish, whose best-selling books include *Eat More, Weigh Less*, published in 1993. When it was first introduced, the Ornish diet eliminated not only meat, chicken, and fish, but also nuts, seeds, avocados, vegetable oils, and even low-fat dairy products. (Today, Ornish permits small amounts of nuts and seeds.)

Among the foods allowed in the original version of the Ornish diet were tortilla chips, pretzels, crackers, and other packaged foods, as long as they were fat-free. The federal government gave a thumbs-up to such products as well. In its Healthy People 2000 goals, released in 1990, the US Department of Health and Human Services called for the food industry to offer at least 5,000 reduced-fat processed foods by the end of the '90s. The industry exceeded that target, flooding the market with low- and no-fat items like salad dressings, chips, ice cream, and of course cookies; SnackWell's became an emblem of the era. These low-fat foods, promoted on the pages of women's and lifestyle magazines as healthy and weight-friendly alternatives to their high-fat counterparts, often had added sugar to compensate for the reduction in fat and contained the same or even more calories.

We all know what happened during this period: While the percentage of calories from fat went down, obesity rates went up, along with the incidence of diabetes. Experts continue to debate the reasons. Some argue that we didn't reduce our fat intake enough. Others say we ate the wrong (i.e., processed) kind of low-fat foods. There's also the fact that calorie intake overall continued to climb.

Whatever the case, one thing is clear: Our society's fat-focused strategy to fight obesity was a big, fat failure and arguably made the problem worse.

Atkins' Answer

Dr. Robert Atkins offered a different explanation for this outcome: We'd pursued the wrong suspect. Fat was innocent, he argued, and the real perpetrators were the pasta, potatoes, and other carbohydrates we were being urged to eat.

The notion that carbs promote weight gain wasn't new. More than a century earlier, William Banting had described his own low-carb weight-loss plan in *Letter on Corpulence, Addressed to the Public.* In this best-selling pamphlet, first published in 1863, the previously obese English undertaker revealed that he had shed 46 pounds by following his doctor's advice to avoid sugar, starch, and "saccharine matter." The first international diet book sensation, it was so popular that *bant* became a verb meaning "to diet."

A 1950s incarnation of the carb-restricted regimen was Dr. Alfred Pennington's DuPont diet, so named because Pennington had prescribed it to overweight employees at the DuPont company. In a 1953 *New England Journal of Medicine* article, Pennington reported that limiting carbohydrates to 1 or 2 percent of calories had "worked out very well" for weight loss because it caused the body to draw on fat stores—a claim familiar to anyone today who follows the keto diet.

The 1960s brought the publication of several low-carb diets, including the best seller *Calories Don't Count*, by Dr. Herman Taller, who was convicted of mail fraud and conspiracy for using the book to promote safflower oil capsules; *The Drinking Man's Diet*, by cosmetics executive Robert Cameron, which allowed all the meat and booze you wanted but no bread or pasta; and *Martinis & Whipped Cream*— how's that for an enticing title?—which included the chapter "Villain Carbohydrates Unmasked."

Atkins, a cardiologist, jumped on the anti-carb bandwagon in the 1960s, and in 1972 published his first book, *Dr. Atkins' Diet Revolution*. Given the 100-year history of carb-shunning, Atkins' prescription for weight loss was hardly revolutionary. But as historian Hillel Schwartz observed, "Each time the diet has reappeared, it has been impervious to its past."

The Atkins diet appeared once again in the 1990s when he released *Dr. Atkins' New Diet Revolution.* Capitalizing on people's dissatisfaction with low-fat diets, Atkins' message that steak and bacon were okay and that bread was bad helped make his book a best seller. Other low-carb diets followed, such as the Zone and South Beach diets. While the diets' regimens differed, all singled out carbohydrates as a contributor to weight gain and restricted them to varying degrees.

Manufacturers of everything from energy bars to ice cream rushed to push out thousands of reformulated products, this time with fewer carbs and more fat. Among those peddling such foods was Atkins himself through his company Atkins Nutritionals. Though Atkins died in 2003, his success at making carbohydrates a dirty word for millions of people continues to this day. He "cast a very long shadow," in the words of *Diet Cults* author Matt Fitzgerald, who asks rhetorically: "Would the gluten-free diet trend or the Paleo Diet have caught fire . . . if Atkins had not first changed the average eater's view of grains?"

MYTH OR TRUTH?

Gluten promotes weight gain.

Gluten, a protein found in wheat, barley, and rye, is harmful for people with celiac disease. While some individuals without celiac disease report symptoms due to gluten (a condition known as gluten sensitivity), it's unproven that weight gain is one of them. In studies, gluten causes body fat to increase in mice, but there haven't been trials demonstrating this in humans. Nor is there proof that gluten-free diets lead to weight loss.

As for the related claim that wheat specifically makes people fat (an idea popularized by the best-selling book *Wheat Belly*), there's again little or no evidence. Wheat has been a staple of diets around the world for centuries without causing obesity, and the notion that today's wheat is more fattening because of selective breeding is scientifically baseless.

Beware of gluten-free versions of breads, crackers, and other foods, which aren't necessarily more healthful or weight friendly. In many cases, they're higher in calories and sugar, and lower in fiber and B vitamins than their gluten-containing counterparts.

Weighing the Diets

Today's anti-carb crusaders, like Dr. David Ludwig and writer Gary Taubes, point to the hormone insulin as key to carbohydrates' alleged evil. Eating high-carb foods boosts insulin production, which they say causes the body to store those calories as fat. This in turn supposedly leads to increased hunger and a slowed metabolism, both of which promote weight gain.

This explanation, which sounds reasonable, is often presented as an established fact. But it's not. Though research by Ludwig appears to support the theory, studies by other investigators do not. For example, when people were fed low-carb diets under carefully controlled conditions, their metabolic rates didn't increase as predicted, but instead barely budged or even *decreased*. And participants lost *less* body fat on a low-carb diet than on a comparable low-fat diet.

What's more, when researchers pooled results from more than 20 observational studies reporting carbohydrate intake, they found no association between higher-carb diets and obesity.

Carb foes say that research refuting their beliefs has design flaws. Yet the fact remains that while they criticize the case against fat for lacking sufficient evidence, their case against carbs suffers from the same weakness.

Pot, meet kettle.

So which side is right? Overall, studies comparing low-fat and low-carb diets suggest neither one.

Consider results from three of the largest trials, all involving overweight or obese adults.·

⮑ A study published in the *New England Journal of Medicine* randomly assigned 811 people to one of four diets, each with a different percentage of calories derived from fat (ranging from 20 to 40 percent), carbohydrates (35 to 65 percent), and protein (15 to 25 percent). After six months, the average weight loss in each group was the same—about 13 pounds. After a year, subjects began to put weight back on. At two years, those who had completed the trial were down about 9 pounds on average from where they had started, with no differences between the lowest-fat and lowest-carb groups.

⮑ An *Annals of Internal Medicine* study involved 307 participants who were assigned to either a low-fat diet (defined as at most 30 percent of calories from fat) or a low-carb diet (20 grams per day for the first three months and then gradually more). After one year, average weight loss (24 pounds) was the same for both diets. After two years, the loss dropped to 15 pounds, and there were still no differences.

⮌ In a study known as DIETFITS, published in the *Journal of the American Medical Association*, 609 subjects were assigned to follow either a healthy low-fat diet (which in practice was 29 percent of calories from fat) or a healthy low-carb diet (30 percent from carbs). For both diets, "healthy" meant maximizing vegetables and whole foods, and minimizing added sugars and refined grains. After one year, people on the two diets shed an average of 12 to 13 pounds, and there were no differences between the groups.

Notice a pattern?

Taken together, these studies show that cutting either fat or carbs can promote weight loss, that weight plateaus and then gradually returns on both diets, and that in the long run—which is what counts—neither holds an advantage.

Other head-to-head comparisons suggest that during the first six months or so, low-carb diets may be more effective, but the difference is relatively small—less than 5 pounds. Such averages obscure the fact that in studies, individual results can vary widely. In the DIETFITS trial, for instance, a few people in each group lost as much as 60 pounds or more, while others gained 20.

Why some people have more success than others on particular diets is unclear. It's possible that genetics may affect who does better on a low-carb or low-fat diet, but the DIETFITS study found no evidence for this. Likewise, insulin status may play a role—some research suggests that low-carb diets are superior for those with insulin resistance or higher insulin levels—but again, DIETFITS failed to show this.

One problem with the research overall is that there's no standard definition of "low" in "low-fat" and "low-carb." For example, for low-fat diets, research usually sets the limit at 30 percent of calories from fat. But some studies use a threshold of 20 percent or lower. Likewise, the upper limit for carbs in studies of low-carb diets ranges from 10 percent of calories to 30 percent or higher.

Proponents of the diets say that if a study doesn't restrict fat or carbs enough, it's not a good test of the diet's effectiveness. Fair point. So how do the most extreme versions of each diet stack up?

Let's start with the Ornish diet, which I described earlier. It limits fat intake to 10 percent of calories—less than a third of what the average American consumes. In two trials comparing Ornish to Atkins and other diets, the Ornish group pared off 5 to 7 pounds after one year, which was either the same as the Atkins group lost or slightly worse, depending on the study.

As for carb-restricted diets, the lowest you can go is keto, short for *ketogenic*. Glucose from carbohydrates is normally our bodies' main source of energy. The keto diet, which has been used for 100 years to treat epilepsy, aims to deprive the body of glucose so that it instead taps stored fat as energy by converting it into compounds called ketones. This typically requires less than 10 percent of calories from carbs, or at most 50 grams of carbs a day—roughly one-fifth of the amount of carbs in the average diet. Going that low means foods such as grains, beans, sweets, starchy vegetables, and most fruits are off-limits.

In a study that pooled results from 13 trials comparing a keto diet to a low-fat diet, the keto diet came out ahead— just barely. After 12 months or longer, subjects on the keto regimen lost 2 pounds more than the low-fat dieters, a difference that the researchers called "of little clinical significance." Translation: meaningless.

Whether a diet restricts fat or carbs, people's adherence typically wanes over time. The longer a study lasts, the more the subjects tend to cheat and overindulge in the "wrong" foods. Dropouts are common, especially for more extreme diets. For example, the aforementioned study of 13 trials testing the keto diet reported that in most of them, at least one-third of the participants quit before the end. In one of the trials, 84 percent failed to make it to the finish line.

If many or most people have trouble sticking with a diet for more than a few months, it doesn't exactly speak well for the diet. But proponents don't see it that way. When low-carb or low-fat diets fail to work as predicted, advocates blame dieters' lack of diligence. And we blame ourselves.

But we shouldn't. Whether the forbidden foods are cheese and chocolate or cereal and corn, highly restrictive diets often leave us feeling deprived. Eliminating foods that we enjoy can do a number on our brains, causing us to crave the foods even more. Sooner or later, most of us yield to temptation. For some dieters, this process can trigger binge eating.

What's more, outlawing entire categories of foods may be bad for our health. For example, the keto diet's lack of whole grains and most fruits, which are key sources of vitamins, minerals, and fiber, can potentially lead to nutrient deficiencies. In addition, replacing carbs with lots of saturated fat can increase LDL, the "bad" cholesterol. (It may also increase HDL—the "good" cholesterol—and decrease harmful blood fats called triglycerides, so the overall effect on heart health is unclear.) Likewise, extremely low-fat diets can pose problems if they contain too little protein and beneficial fat from sources such as oils, nuts, and fatty fish.

While severely restricting fat or carbs can be an effective strategy in some cases, it's not a magic bullet and doesn't work long term for most people. The truth is that there's no single "best" diet for everyone. Yet diet peddlers have a financial incentive to keep us hoping and believing otherwise. So do researchers who get funding and career advancement for churning out more futile studies that look to crown a "winner" in the low-carb versus low-fat versus low-whatever wars. In fact, there are no winners. There are only losers—us—for being led down this pointless and potentially harmful path.

Jordan's Journey

Jordan was searching for a way to shed pounds but found himself lost in a sea of diet options. Then, in 2012, having just graduated from college, he stumbled upon a book that touted the keto diet. It broke through the noise with what seemed like a dieter's dream: Eat as much fat as you want—bacon, cheese, and steak included—on one simple condition: no carbs.

Jordan, who had been overweight for most of his life, liked going to the gym but had trouble controlling his eating. Working at a restaurant helped him pay for school but also contributed to his challenges with food.

Jordan hoped the keto diet would provide a solution. It didn't take long, though, for him to hit some major speed bumps. Without carbs, he felt his energy to be noticeably diminished. The workouts he used to enjoy became draining attempts to push himself. "I was always hitting a wall," he says. At gatherings with friends and family, he felt guilt and embarrassment over his efforts to carb-proof the menu.

What's more, the weight wasn't coming off as he had expected. Every time he lost a few pounds, they would reappear even more quickly. Over a two-year period, Jordan tried keto on and off for a total of about eight months. During that time, his attempts at weight loss were further derailed by his new career in data analytics, which came with lots of business travel and social drinking.

Jordan's disappointing results and deepening frustration finally prompted him to dump the keto diet altogether. Thinking that there had to be something better, he resumed his search and eventually discovered what he'd been looking for—but it wasn't another restrictive diet. Instead of shunning certain nutrients or foods, he focused on the overall makeup of his diet, paying attention to what and how much he put in his body.

Thanks to his new eating habits, which supply all the nutrients he needs, Jordan has had more effective workouts. And he's lost 40 pounds, weight that he has managed by and large to keep off.

MYTH OR TRUTH?

You should avoid carbs that have a high glycemic index.

The glycemic index (GI), which ranges from 0 to 100, ranks carbohydrate-containing foods on how much they raise blood sugar. Champions of the scale claim that high-GI carbs such as potatoes promote weight gain more than low-GI carbs like beans. (A related concept, glycemic load, or GL, takes into account both GI and the amount of carbohydrate per serving.) But studies overall have failed to show that low-GI or -GL diets are superior for weight loss. And the concept of GI itself is flawed because it assumes that foods are consumed in isolation on an empty stomach, which often isn't the case. Eating fat along with a high-GI food, for example, suppresses blood sugar spikes. In addition, other variables, such as cooking methods and ripeness, can affect a food's impact on blood sugar, and responses can vary from person to person. So GI is often an unreliable guide.

Souring on Sugar

Yet another nominee for the title of Most Villainous is sugar, and the person most responsible for conferring that honor is Dr. Robert Lustig. In 2009, he gave a lecture titled "Sugar: The Bitter Truth," in which he called sugar a "poison" that's the main cause of obesity and other health problems. A video of the talk, which was posted on YouTube, has attracted more than 10 million views.

Lustig has also published a best-selling book that elaborates on his theory about sugar's role. Titled *Fat Chance*, the book labels sugar—or, to be more exact, fructose, a component of refined sugar, high-fructose corn syrup, and other caloric sweeteners—a "toxin" and "the primary . . . villain, the Darth Vader of the Empire, beckoning you to the dark side."

Sugar is a 50-50 mixture of glucose and fructose, each of which the body processes differently. When we consume glucose or other carbohydrates, our insulin levels rise, which prompts the hormone leptin to signal to our brains that we're full. (More on leptin in the next chapter.) But fructose doesn't bump up insulin production, so according to Lustig, the brain doesn't get the message we're full, and we keep eating,

Another difference is that unlike glucose, which cells throughout the body can use as fuel, fructose is metabolized almost exclusively by the liver. Lustig says when we consume more fructose than the liver can handle, the excess wreaks metabolic havoc, contributing to fat production, insulin resistance, and abnormal cholesterol, among other things.

In studies of rodents, large amounts of fructose bring on obesity and other effects Lustig describes. But the animals usually receive much higher doses of fructose than we typically consume. Plus, rodents metabolize fructose differently than humans do, so the relevance of this research is questionable.

Overall, human studies don't support Lustig's theory, at least when it comes to weight. Take, for example, the many trials in which researchers fed participants diets containing fructose and, for comparison purposes, slashed the fructose and replaced it with other carbohydrates while keeping total calories the same. A study commissioned by the

World Health Organization that pooled results from such trials concluded that the higher-fructose diets were no more fattening than the lower-fructose ones.

The WHO study also showed a link between higher sugar intake and higher weight. But this and other research suggests that these extra pounds are due to extra calories from sugar, not to anything uniquely villainous about fructose or sugar.

As for the claim that sugar is the main cause of obesity, consider recent trends: Between 2003 and 2016, total sugar intake among adults in the US *declined* by 17 percent. During the same period, adult obesity rates *rose* by 23 percent. If sugar were guilty as charged, you'd expect to see obesity rates falling—or at least not climbing.

None of this is to say that eating lots of sugar is okay. While there's no hard proof that it's the only or even the leading cause of obesity, excess sugar does contribute to weight gain, diabetes, and other health problems, and most of us take in too much of it. The fact that it's not *the* problem doesn't mean it's not *a* problem.

But when fructose specifically and sugar generally become enemy No. 1, there are unintended consequences. For starters, we now see lots of foods and beverages proudly proclaiming themselves to be free of high-fructose corn syrup (HFCS). In fact, the name is misleading; HFCS is not really high in fructose. Like sugar, it's roughly 50 percent fructose (or less), and there's no solid evidence that HFCS is any worse for us than sugar—a point that even Lustig acknowledges. Yet by labeling products "HFCS-free," manufacturers may fool us into thinking that such foods are less fattening or healthier, even though they're loaded with sugar or other caloric sweeteners.

In addition, the vilification of sugar has led to an explosion of low- and no-sugar processed foods, which mirrors what we've seen with low-fat and low-carb foods. Typically manufacturers replace the sugar with artificial sweeteners, and as I discuss in the next chapter, there's limited evidence that these foods promote weight loss. Some research has even linked them to weight *gain* along with other negative health effects, including diabetes. If we overconsume these sugar-restricted foods as we have other enemy-free foods, this antidote to the "poison" sugar won't shrink our waistlines and could very well end up further fueling the flames of obesity and related conditions.

MYTH OR TRUTH?

Fruit is fattening.

Like foods with added sugar, fruit contains a combination of fructose and glucose, with one serving delivering as many as 20 grams of sugar or more in some cases. But fruit also contains fiber, which slows the absorption of sugar. In addition, the fiber and water in fruit help fill us up so we're less likely to eat too much of it (though there are exceptions, like dried fruit). Overall, research shows that fruit does not contribute to weight gain and is even linked to weight loss. And low-sugar fruits aren't necessarily better for your waistline than high-sugar ones. In three large studies, apples and pears, whose sugar content is on the high side, were more strongly associated with weight loss than lower-sugar fruits like grapefruit.

Fruit juice is a different story, however. Stripped of fiber, it typically has more sugar and calories than fruit and is less filling. Research has linked it to weight *gain*. All reasons why it's better to eat your fruit than drink it. (For more on fruit, see chapter 4.)

Drink Yourself Fat?

In recent years, the anti-sugar spotlight has turned increasingly to soda and other sugar-sweetened beverages (SSBs), such as fruit drinks, sports drinks, and energy drinks. Some public health and obesity experts have singled out SSBs as a contributor to obesity because the drinks are a major source of liquid calories and added sugar in our diets, and fill us up less than solid foods. Groups with higher consumption of SSBs, such as African Americans and Hispanics, have higher obesity rates.

In 2009, New York City's health department launched an anti-SSB campaign that drew national attention to the issue. Called "Pouring on the Pounds," it included ads in subways showing congealed fat being poured from a soda bottle with the tagline "Don't drink yourself fat." Even more unappetizing was a video in which a man scarfed down globs of fat from a soda can as they fell down his chin. That was followed by text stating that "drinking 1 can of soda a day can make you 10 pounds fatter a year"—a claim that was challenged at the time by some experts at the NYC health department and elsewhere.

As for what studies show about SSBs and weight, it depends on whom you ask and where their funding comes from. A study examining 17 large reviews of evidence found that those with funding from industry (such as soda sellers) tended to report that the research is inconclusive. But reviews with no reported conflicts of interest usually concluded that there is an association between SSBs and weight gain or obesity.

If SSBs do promote weight gain—which is likely—the impact may be relatively small. A team of Harvard researchers who have no industry ties estimated that each added daily serving of SSBs (e.g., going from one to two sodas a day) is associated with an average weight increase in adults of less than ½ pound per year.

Recent trends also cast doubt on the notion that SSBs are a leading cause of obesity. As with total sugar intake, consumption of SSBs has decreased in recent years. Between 2003 and 2016, calorie intake from SSBs plummeted by nearly 50 percent, with SSBs accounting for around 4 percent of total calories in adults and 5 percent in kids by 2016. During this time, the proportion of people who never drink SSBs increased while the percentage of heavy users declined substantially.

Recall what happened with obesity during the same period: Rates continued their march upward, from 32 percent to nearly 40 percent among adults. Obesity rates among youth also rose. As with sugar, consumption and obesity trends should be going in the same direction, not the opposite one, if in fact SSBs are a major driver of the obesity epidemic.

Despite the limited evidence for SSBs' role, many obesity experts and a handful of cities have embraced the idea of taxing SSBs as a way to slow or reverse the epidemic. Supporters often compare sugary beverages to tobacco, arguing that SSB taxes can cut down people's consumption and weight just as tobacco taxes have reduced smoking.

While research does show that taxes can decrease purchases of SSBs, there's no hard evidence that this leads to weight loss. Perhaps that's because unlike tobacco, SSBs can be replaced with any number of alternatives.

To be sure, someone who opts against soda may go for water. But the person may be just as likely to choose a beverage such as fruit juice, chocolate milk, or beer, all of which can have as many calories as soda or more. Or an individual may instead buy something to eat, like a candy bar or potato chips. In short, there's no guarantee that discouraging SSBs will result in more weight-friendly purchases.

Given that emotions tend to run high around SSB taxes, I should make it clear where I'm coming from: Because soda and other SSBs aren't healthful, I don't drink them. I have no ties, financial or otherwise, to any industry related to SSBs. Nor do I view the issue through a conservative political lens.

My concern is the harm that SSB taxes can do to our efforts to combat obesity. Supporters of a tax sometimes say, "Well, it can't hurt." But that's not true. When, despite a lack of evidence, measures like SSB taxes are promoted for weight loss and then fail to deliver, scientists' and public health officials' credibility can take a beating. That's especially a problem given the distrust of scientific authority that already exists among a growing number of people. Broken promises could make it harder to win support for future anti-obesity measures, even if they have strong scientific backing.

An even bigger downside is that all the time and effort devoted to fighting for SSB taxes is time and effort *not* spent on things that matter far more, like the overall composition of our diets. Taxing SSBs is a politically charged and difficult struggle, and even proponents now acknowledge that this approach alone won't curb obesity. It makes little sense to use limited resources (whether expertise, attention, or money) to wage an uphill battle that's unlikely to have much, if any, impact. Whether the crusade occurs in scientific journals or before city councils, it's misplaced effort that could be much more effective if directed elsewhere.

MYTH OR TRUTH?

Beer and other types of alcohol give you a beer belly.

Alcohol has 7 calories per gram—nearly twice the number supplied by carbohydrates and protein. This is often cited as a reason that drinking supposedly packs on pounds. But in fact, studies generally show that light to moderate consumption of beer, wine, and other alcoholic beverages is *not* associated with weight gain or more fat around the waist. What's more, non-overweight women who drink moderately may be *less* likely to gain weight and become obese than teetotalers, according to some research. But heavy drinking (meaning three or more drinks a day) and binge drinking are linked to obesity and belly fat, especially in men. Watch out for mixed drinks with added sugar and calories, which may promote weight gain more than alcohol-only beverages.

The Elephant in the Room

In the ancient parable "The Blind Men and the Elephant," a group of unsighted men who have never encountered an elephant try to figure out what it is by touching it. Each man feels a different part of the animal from trunk to tail and reaches a different conclusion. In some versions of the story, the disagreeing men come to blows.

Nutrition expert Dr. David Katz uses this story to highlight what he calls the *ONAAT fallacy*, which stands for "one nutrient at a time." When we fixate on individual components of the diet, whether fat, carbs, gluten, fructose, or whatever else, we miss the big picture and fail to see the elephant in the room. Yes, too many hamburgers or too much bread or too much soda may contribute to obesity, but none of these alone is the cause.

Instead of focusing on individual villains, we need to pay attention to the general quality of our diets. This means emphasizing whole foods like vegetables, fruits, whole grains, beans, nuts, seafood, and lean poultry, and minimizing highly processed foods (sometimes called "ultra-processed" foods) such as chips, cookies, refined grains, soda, hot dogs, and fries. Research suggests that this eating pattern is effective for not only managing weight long term but also optimizing our health.

Such an approach provides lots of leeway. There's no list of foods that you *must* eat. Nor are there "evil" foods that you can't ever touch. The idea is to think broadly about your diet and opt for whole foods over highly processed ones as much as possible. You can accomplish this with countless combinations of foods and varying proportions of fats, carbohydrates, and protein.

As for why emphasizing whole foods may help control weight, research is still emerging, but they tend to be less energy dense (meaning fewer calories per ounce) than highly processed ones, they're typically higher in fiber and more filling, and we often eat them more slowly, giving our brains time to get the message that we've had enough. It's also possible that whole and highly processed foods may have different effects on appetite-related hormones, as well as on bacteria in the gut that affect the absorption of calories from food. (See chapter 2 for more on the role of gut bacteria.)

Focusing on your overall dietary pattern also increases the likelihood that you can find ways to eat that don't leave you feeling deprived. That's crucial because, as previously discussed, villain-driven diets that forbid lists of foods you enjoy typically aren't sustainable over the long term and can even cause harm.

Though self-deprivation and sacrifice are not virtues when it comes to weight control, these principles are deeply rooted in diet culture—a fact that helps explain the appeal of declaring certain foods off-limits. Likewise, our never-ending quest for quick fixes draws us to promises that simply banishing bad guys—whether fat, carbs, meat, beans, wheat, sugar, or something else—will solve the problem.

The food industry has made this solution seem even easier by churning out more and more convenience foods that are free of every conceivable villain. But our embrace of these ostensibly beneficial foods has likely made our struggle with weight harder. That's because most are highly processed—the kinds of foods that we should be eating fewer of, not more, for long-term weight control. In such a way, our attempt to exorcise dietary demons, aided and abetted by the food industry, has blown up in our faces.

The real offenders, it turns out, are all those who mislead us about villains—and all of us who keep falling for their false promises.

What to Do

⊃ While a diet that bans certain foods may be an effective kick-starter for some people, don't count on it to work long term. Instead, focus on your overall eating pattern, emphasizing vegetables, fruits, beans, nuts, seeds, seafood, lean poultry, and whole grains such as oats and brown rice. (To spot whole-grain foods, check the ingredient label; the word *whole* should be listed first.)

⊃ Minimize highly processed foods including refined grains (such as white bread), chips, cookies, hot dogs, bacon, fried foods, and sugary beverages. (One clue: A long list of ingredients on the label.) You don't need to banish such items from your diet. Just limit portions and make them occasional treats rather than regular staples.

⮂ Don't try to overhaul your eating habits all at once. Make gradual changes and be patient; it takes time to adjust to a healthier diet.

Chapter 2

THE CALORIE FALLACY

You can say one thing for Professor Mark Haub: He knows how to make a lesson stick.

Haub, who teaches nutrition at Kansas State University, wanted to prove to his students that weight loss is simply about calories. So, for 10 weeks, the portly professor proceeded to eat an 1,800-calorie diet consisting of a Twinkie every three hours. He also dined on Doritos, Little Debbies, sugary cereal, and other junk food.

When he started, Haub tipped the scales at 201 pounds, which for his height was considered overweight. By the end of his snack-food spree, he had lost 27 pounds, putting him at a svelte 174.

The story went viral, with the media dubbing Haub's eating plan the Twinkie Diet. Undoubtedly some who heard the news eagerly stocked up on the spongy yellow snacks. But Haub's intention wasn't to urge people to eat more Twinkies. The point, he said, was that he had consumed 800 fewer calories daily than the number needed to maintain his weight. In other words, the key to weight control is counting calories: If you take in fewer than you burn, you lose weight. It's that simple.

Haub's message has been standard advice for more than a century. Its most influential early champion was Lulu Hunt Peters, a physician and syndicated newspaper columnist who popularized the notion of calories in her 1918 best-selling book, *Diet and Health, with Key to the Calories*.

Peters, who had struggled with her own weight, advised readers how many calories they should consume and how many were contained in various foods—both relatively novel concepts at the time. "Hereafter," she wrote, "you are going to eat calories of food. Instead of saying one slice of bread, or a piece of pie, you will say 100 calories of bread, 350 calories of pie."

Foreshadowing the Twinkie Diet, she wrote: "You may eat just what you like—candy, pie, cake, fat meat, butter, cream—but count your calories!"

Today leading health authorities have a similarly calorie-centric view of weight control. For example, the National Institutes of Health (NIH) website says that excess weight results "when you take in more calories than you use." Likewise, the World Health Organization explains that the "fundamental cause of obesity and overweight is an energy imbalance between calories consumed and calories expended." And the USDA's Nutrition.gov site advises that "weight loss can be achieved by either eating fewer calories or by burning more calories with physical activity."

According to these and other experts, it all boils down to straightforward math: Calories in minus calories out. (More on the "calories out" part in the next chapter.) Countless millions who struggle with their weight heed this message, dutifully tracking their calorie intake. But eventually many discover that all the counting is in vain. That's because while calories matter, they're not the whole story.

Saying that weight control can be boiled down to calorie counts is like saying your risk of a heart attack can be boiled down to your cholesterol score. It's overly simplistic. Yes, cholesterol is relevant, but so are other factors, such as age, gender, activity level, blood pressure, and genetics.

The same is true for calories. Other factors, including metabolism, digestion, and genetics, play a role in how many calories your body craves and how it absorbs and burns the calories you consume.

While counting calories can work in the short term, it typically leads to frustration and failure in the long run. Had Professor Haub's Twinkie stunt lasted a couple of years instead of a couple of months, the outcome—and his lesson—would likely have been far different.

Burn, Baby (Carrot), Burn

Before I elaborate on the problems with calorie counting, let's briefly consider what, exactly, a calorie is.

In chemistry, the calorie is a unit of thermal energy. One calorie is the amount of energy required to raise the temperature of 1 gram of water by 1 degree Celsius. So what does this have to do with food?

To measure the energy in food, 19th-century scientists used contraptions called bomb calorimeters, in which a sealed chamber containing food was immersed in water and the food set on fire and burned to a crisp. The resulting increase in water temperature was measured in—you guessed it—calories. (Technically, the unit of measure was a kilocalorie, but today we typically shorten it to "calorie" when referring to kilocalories in food.)

A shortcoming of bomb calorimeters is that they don't exactly replicate what happens in the human body. When we eat, some of the calories we take in aren't absorbed; they're used to digest food or lost in feces and urine.

To get more accurate estimates of calories consumed and used, Wilbur Atwater—a Wesleyan University chemist who's been called the "first modern nutrition scientist"— built a calorimeter in the 1890s that was large enough to house people.

The device, which consisted of a chamber surrounded by water, measured how much heat subjects gave off as they ate, slept, and did other activities over the course of several days. In addition, subjects' feces were collected and burned in a bomb calorimeter to determine how much energy the excrement contained (a decidedly crappy job that Atwater presumably assigned to some lucky research assistant).

Atwater's intention wasn't to help people lose weight. It was, in a sense, just the opposite: to show how American workers could get the most calories from the least amount of food and thereby save money for themselves, their employ- ers, and society. To that end, Atwater pulled together results from his own work and that of others to calculate calorie values for proteins, fats, and carbohydrates. Atwater's fig- ures—4 calories per gram for protein, 9 calories per gram for fat, and 4 calories per gram for carbohydrate—became known as "Atwater factors" and remain the basis today for measuring calorie counts of foods and beverages.

Calorie Miscounts

When you come across a calorie value for, say, a box of cook- ies at the store or a burger at a restaurant, it's pretty safe to assume that the company didn't burn any feces or force any- one into a calorimeter. Instead, they likely used a nutrient database to determine the calories of various constituents in the food and then added up the numbers.

But counts aren't always accurate. In fact, the Food and Drug Administration (FDA) allows numbers on nutri- tion labels to be off by as much as 20 percent, and usually the error is an undercount. That means, for example, that ice cream claiming to have 180 calories per serving may actually have 215. Making matters worse is the widespread problem of unrealistic serving sizes. With ice cream, if you eat a cup (a normal amount) rather than 2/3 cup (the usual serving size), you could be getting as many as 325 calories instead of the 180 listed on the label.

Calorie counts for restaurant foods can be even more misleading. In a study of more than 200 foods from fast-food and sit-down restaurants, about 1 in 5 items contained at least 100 calories per serving over the listed amount. The 13 worst offenders had, on average, 52 percent more calories than advertised, and one dish packed more than triple the stated number, which translated to a 1,000-calorie surplus surprise. As with calories on food labels, the FDA doesn't systematically check calorie figures on menus for accuracy, so there's little to stop sellers from providing incorrect counts.

Listed calories may also be wrong because of the way our bodies digest certain foods. Take almonds, for instance. Nutrition labels show them to have up to 170 calories per ounce. But the Atwater factors upon which this number is based don't take into account that almonds pass through the intestines partly undigested. As a result, the body doesn't absorb all 170 calories. The actual count, according to research, is 129—a sizable difference. Studies have found listed calories for other nuts such as walnuts and cashews to be overstated as well.

Whether foods are cooked can also affect how many calories we absorb from them. In studies, when mice ate meat and starchy foods that were cooked, they lost less weight than when consuming the same foods raw. What these results demonstrate—beyond a possible weight-loss regimen for mice—is that cooking and processing can make foods more digestible and thereby increase their usable calories. Calorie counts often don't reflect this fact and may be too high for some uncooked or unprocessed foods.

Then there's the issue of insoluble fiber, a.k.a. roughage, which is in foods such as bran, whole wheat bread, beans, and vegetables. This type of fiber is not digested and passes through the body. Whether we absorb any calories from it is a matter of debate. In the US, manufacturers are allowed to subtract the grams of insoluble fiber, at 4 calories per gram, when calculating calorie totals. In Canada, though, insoluble fiber is only partly subtracted, using a formula of 2 calories per gram. The result is that the same food can have different calorie counts on the label depending on whether it's purchased in Detroit or Toronto.

What all this means is that we shouldn't take calorie counts as gospel. Yet too often that's how we view them, a notion that's reinforced by their appearance in big, bold text at the very top of every food nutrition label. This endows the numbers with an unduly exalted status and a false appearance of precision.

MYTH OR TRUTH?

Some foods have "negative" calories.

Foods such as celery, cucumbers, and lettuce have gained a reputation as weight-loss aids because they supposedly require more calories to digest than they provide. It's true that the body uses energy to digest and metabolize food. But the calories expended for this—known as the thermic effect of food—do not exceed the calories in the food itself, even for very low-calorie foods such as celery.

Ice-cold water is a different story. It has no calories, and we burn a few calories to warm it up to body temperature. But the number is likely too small to have an impact on our weight.

Unreliable Estimates

Accurate or not, calorie counts aren't available for everything we eat, so we sometimes have to rely on our own estimates. And according to research, these numbers are notoriously unreliable. For example, in a survey of 2,200 adults, consumers' guesses about calories in popular restaurant foods ranging from pancakes to onion rings undershot the reality by an average of 165 calories. Some missed not just the mark but the entire target. For example, consumers put the calorie count for a 12-ounce daiquiri at 284; the actual figure was 674. For a beef taco salad, the average guess was 446 calories. The real count: 906, a difference of more than 450 calories.

Unconscious biases can further skew our calorie estimates. For instance, there's the "health halo" bias, which makes us more likely to underestimate calories in foods that are marketed as healthful. When researchers asked 115 mall shoppers to taste paired samples of cookies, chips, and yogurt, participants judged the items labeled "organic" to be lower in calories than those foods' conventional counterparts. In fact, the foods in each pair—and their calorie counts—were identical.

Similarly, adding a healthful side dish to a meal tends to lower consumers' calorie guesstimates. For example, in a study in which subjects were shown either a cheeseburger alone or a cheeseburger paired with a salad, they judged the burger-salad combo to have *fewer* calories than just the cheeseburger. Researchers refer to this type of error as "averaging bias," which happens when we combine a healthy and an unhealthy item. Because the combination seems more healthful, our brains may trick us into subtracting calories.

Now, if you're questioning the intelligence of those who make such mistakes, you shouldn't. The inability to estimate calories correctly doesn't mean that they (or you) are stupid. Instead, it's a reflection of how exceedingly difficult the task is. Calories are an abstract concept—we can't see, feel, or taste them—so it's no surprise that our judgments about them are prone to error.

Even if you're in the small minority of people who *can* accurately figure out how many calories they're consuming, you've won just half the battle. The other half is knowing how many you burn and therefore need to take in to achieve a negative energy balance for weight loss. Here, too, our estimates tend to be woefully inadequate. In a survey of 1,000 people by the International Food Information Council Foundation, about half of respondents said they had no idea how many calories they burned each day. And when asked the number they needed, 85 percent of those who responded either guessed incorrectly or said they didn't know.

Online calculators can tell you how many calories you expend each day, but it's at best an approximation. Wearable devices are also an option, but research shows that their results are unreliable. Arriving at an accurate number is difficult because the calculation is complex, involving how much energy we need for basic functions like breathing and circulation at rest (known as basal metabolic rate, or BMR); how much we burn during everyday activities and exercise; and how much through digesting food (the thermic effect of food). A host of other factors, including age, gender, weight, and body fat, play a role.

Given all the challenges of accurately calculating how many calories we need and how many we consume, it's unreasonable to expect counting calories to be effective as a weight-loss strategy. Even nutrition experts Marion Nestle and Malden Nesheim, who make a case for the importance of calories in their book titled *Why Calories Count*, advise against counting them "because it is too difficult to do precisely."

Battling Biology

The difficulty is reason enough to shun calorie counting. But there's also an even bigger problem: Tallying calories fails to take into account other variables that can affect how much we weigh.

As we reduce calories and lose weight, biological changes kick in to preserve body fat and protect us from starvation. One such adaptation is a change in metabolism. The body of a lighter person has a lower BMR than that of a heavier person. As we shed pounds, we burn even fewer calories than expected for a person of our reduced size—a phenomenon that scientists call *adaptive thermogenesis*. In essence, our bodies become more fuel efficient, making it increasingly difficult to shed more pounds and to maintain weight loss with the same number of calories. Unfortunately, this evolutionary gift, designed to keep us alive in times of scarcity, isn't something we can switch off or send back when we don't need it.

We also get pushback from various hormones regulating appetite. Among these is leptin, whose name is derived from the Greek word for "thin." Produced by the body's fat cells, leptin tells an area of the brain known as the hypothalamus how much fat we have stored. When we restrict calories and lose weight, leptin levels decrease, signaling to the brain that we need to eat more. The result is an uptick in hunger.

Another key hormone is ghrelin, known as the hunger hormone. Released mainly by the stomach when we haven't eaten, it acts on the hypothalamus to crank up appetite. Ghrelin levels also rise when we're shedding pounds, and research shows that the hormone stays elevated for at least a year after weight loss. Likewise, leptin levels remain depressed after weight loss.

These and other hormones are part of the body's intricate feedback mechanisms controlling hunger, fullness, metabolism, and fat storage. Though scientists don't fully understand all the mechanisms, one thing is certain: our weight hinges on highly complex biological processes that entail far more than how many calories we consciously choose to consume.

MYTH OR TRUTH?

A 3,500-calorie deficit equals 1 pound of fat.

You may have heard the often-repeated rule of thumb that to lose 1 pound, you need to consume 3,500 fewer calories than you burn. But this is misleading. Based on 1950s research in overweight women, the simplistic formula fails to take individual differences into account or to consider how the body adapts to weight loss. As a result, it typically overestimates how much a person will lose. For example, according to the rule, if you burn 100 calories a day more than you take in, you should drop 50 pounds over five years. But other estimates, which recognize that BMR declines as we get lighter, put the reduction at closer to 10 pounds. And that assumes you're able to resist the strong biological urge to eat more.

Skinny Genes

Our genetic makeup also affects weight regulation. As evidence, look no further than those maddening people who seemingly can eat whatever they want and never gain an ounce. Conventional wisdom has it that such individuals are blessed with "good genes," and research shows that genes do affect how our bodies respond to calories.

In one study, researchers locked up 12 pairs of male identical twins in a college dormitory for four months, supervising their every move. (Yes, the twins agreed to this!) The subjects were fed 1,000 calories a day more than their normal intake, and physical activity was limited. As you would expect, they gained weight. But the amount varied, ranging from about 10 to 30 pounds. What's more, the difference in the amount of weight gained was much smaller between twins in a pair than among different twin pairs. In other words, twins in each pair experienced relatively similar increases in weight, suggesting that genetic factors influence how easily we gain.

The same goes for weight loss. In a study of 14 pairs of obese female twins, the volunteers were housed in a hospital and fed a very low-calorie diet for a month. As with the study in male twins, changes in weight differed fairly widely among subjects. What was striking was how those changes were distributed: There was far more similarity in weight loss within pairs than between pairs.

Taken together, these two studies tell us that when calories are cut (or increased) by a specific amount, the change in weight will vary from person to person, and these differences are due at least in part to genetics.

Further evidence comes from population studies, which show that certain groups of people are more prone to obesity than others. For example, in the US, African Americans,

Native Americans, and Pacific Islanders are more likely to be obese than Caucasians, and Asian Americans are less likely. Obviously, a complex mix of factors beyond genetics, including diet, lifestyle, socioeconomic status, and discrimination, may account for these differences, and determining the exact contribution of each is impossible. But gene-mapping studies in people with mixed racial heritage, including African Americans and Native Americans, have found that those with a greater percentage of European ancestry are less likely to be overweight or obese. This suggests that genetics does indeed contribute to the greater tendency among some populations to carry excess weight.

There's no single "fat gene," however. In fact, there are thought to be hundreds of weight-related genes, which affect everything from appetite and cravings to metabolism and fat storage. One theory is that some people have so-called thrifty genes, which allow them to store fat more easily. In previous eras, these genes were beneficial because they enabled people to survive the famines that were a regular part of life. But now, in an age when food is always readily available for most people, thrifty genes are a disadvantage because they increase susceptibility to being overweight or obese.

The Pima Indians of Arizona are a frequently cited example of this phenomenon. When exposed to a modern lifestyle, more than two-thirds of Pimas became obese. By contrast, Pimas living in a remote area of Mexico, where they maintained their traditional subsistence lifestyle, had relatively low rates of obesity.

Not all scientists buy the thrifty genes hypothesis, and it alone can't account for recent trends in overweight and obesity. Nevertheless, it may help explain why some individuals and groups are more likely than others to put on weight and to have trouble losing it.

Gut Reaction

Yet another possible contributor to weight is the mix of microbes in our gut. This community of bacteria, viruses, and other microorganisms, known as the microbiota, helps break down food and extract energy from it. Studies show that the microbiota of obese people differs from that of lean individuals. Those who are heavy tend to have a less diverse array of microbes and a higher percentage of bacteria known as Firmicutes, which cause more calories to be absorbed from food than do other bacteria.

To show how gut microbes contribute to weight gain, scientists transplanted the microbiota of obese and lean mice into mice whose guts contained no bacteria. Though the mice all ate the same amount of food, those receiving microbiota from obese mice became fatter than those given microbes from lean mice.

In another experiment—skip this if you're eating—lean, bacteria-free mice were fed feces from human twins. One twin in each pair was obese and the other lean. Mice receiving the fat twins' poop became fat, while those given lean people's feces remained lean. The mice that bulked up consumed the same number of calories as the thin mice.

There's anecdotal evidence of a similar phenomenon in people. When the stool of an overweight teenager was transplanted into the gut of her mother—a method used to treat recurrent infections of the bacterium *Clostridium difficile*, or *C. diff*—the mother quickly gained more than 30 pounds and became obese. Prior to the transplant, the mother's weight had remained close to normal.

Though research on the relationship between microbiota and weight is still in its infancy, it suggests that two people can eat the same amount of the same food and experience different effects on their weight depending on the makeup of their microbiota. Those whose gut microbes harvest more energy from food may be more likely to pack on pounds because it's the calories we absorb—as opposed to the ones we ingest—that matter when it comes to our weight.

MYTH OR TRUTH?

Medications can cause weight gain.

An unwelcome side effect of certain medicines is that they can slow metabolism, cause fluid retention, increase fat storage, or stimulate appetite, all of which may lead to weight gain. The amount of weight varies from person to person. Here are some common types of drugs known to increase weight:

- ➲ Antidepressants, including types known as SSRIs and tricyclic antidepressants

- ➲ Antihistamines

- ➲ Blood pressure medicines known as beta-blockers

- ➲ Diabetes medications, including insulin

- ➲ Mood stabilizers, such as lithium

- ➲ Steroid hormones, such as prednisone

Not every drug in each category triggers weight gain, and not everyone is affected. As for other potential culprits, many women report that birth control pills cause them to put on weight, though studies have generally failed to prove this. Antibiotics have long been used to fatten farm animals, and it's thought that the drugs may have a similar effect in people by altering gut microbes. Research has linked antibiotic use to higher weights in children, but there's less evidence about the impact on adults.

The Diet Soda Paradox

Perhaps no food illustrates the shortcomings of calorie math more than diet soda. The logic behind the beverages seems, on the surface, unassailable: They have virtually no calories, and fewer calories mean fewer pounds, so switching to diet drinks is an effective way to lose weight.

It's a message we've heard for many years. As far back as the 1960s, ad campaigns for Tab urged women to drink the diet beverage to remain slim and attractive to their husbands. "Have a shape he can't forget," said one of the TV commercials, which featured a thin, young woman flitting about in a short tennis dress.

The blatantly sexist nature of these ads wasn't the only problem. It turns out their claim that diet soda helps control your weight was unproven. And more than 50 years and hundreds of studies later, it's still unproven.

As a whole, research has failed to show that consuming diet sodas and artificially sweetened foods leads to weight loss. Though some studies (often funded by the artificial sweetener industry) have found a benefit, independent studies have generally concluded that diet sodas have no effect on weight. And in some research, artificially sweetened beverages and foods have been linked to weight *gain*.

As for why diet sodas don't appear to have their intended effect, one theory is that they mess with our brains. When we drink them, our taste receptors signal that we're getting sugar. But since the expected calories don't materialize, the body's hormonal responses go haywire, increasing appetite and prompting us to eat more.

Another possibility is that diet soda affects the mix of microbes in the gut, leading to a harmful imbalance. But only certain artificial sweeteners appear to alter gut microbiota, and research in humans is limited.

Whatever the reason or reasons that diet soda fails to control weight, its drawbacks don't end there. Research has associated it with a host of health problems, including diabetes, dementia, heart disease, strokes, and premature death. While these studies don't prove cause and effect—diet soda drinkers might have behaviors or traits not taken into account that increase their health risks—the research raises the real possibility that the quest to cut calories with diet soda is having harmful effects.

On the Menu: Unintended Consequences

To further understand the unintended consequences of calorie fixation, consider what's happened with restaurant menus. In the US, the law requires calorie counts to be posted by all outlets that sell prepared foods or beverages and have 20 or more locations. As previously mentioned, people tend to do a poor job of estimating calories in foods. Menu listings are intended to attack the obesity epidemic by arming consumers with information and thereby prompting them to select lower-calorie foods.

But it hasn't worked out that way. While some research in lab settings has found calorie information to have a beneficial effect, most real-world studies have not. Pooling results from 14 relatively rigorous studies, researchers concluded that menu labeling does not reduce the number of calories ordered or consumed. Other research shows that people with higher obesity rates who might benefit most, including those with less education and lower incomes, are least likely to notice or use calorie information.

There's even some evidence that labeling leads people to order foods with *more* calories. It could be that when some individuals see, for example, a count of 500 calories for a large order of fries, coupled with a 2,000-calorie-per-day recommendation, they give themselves permission to order the item because its calories are well below the daily limit. Without this information, they might have been more likely to skip the fries.

Another possible effect is that menu counts may promote or exacerbate eating disorders in some people. In a study of 1,800 young men and women, the use of menu listings to limit calories was highest among those who engaged in unhealthy eating behaviors such as skipping meals, purging, or taking laxatives or diet pills.

Perhaps the most common problem is that when people do consult calorie counts to guide their choices, they may be steered toward foods that aren't optimal for weight loss and health. Let's say, for example, you're grabbing breakfast at Starbucks and considering whether to go with a cinnamon raisin bagel or a spinach wrap. The bagel has 20 fewer calories, so by that metric, it's a better choice. But in fact, it's not. The bagel's refined grains make it a highly processed food—the type, as discussed in chapter 1, that's more likely to leave you feeling hungry after you eat it. The wrap, which in addition to spinach includes tomatoes, egg whites, and feta cheese, is more filling and provides far more nutrients. In short, though the wrap has more calories, it's a better option when it comes to your weight and your health.

Relying on calorie counts may compel us to choose other highly processed items, such as baked chips instead of nuts, a hot dog rather than a salad, or a fudge bar instead of fruit. Fixating on calorie measurements takes the focus off the overall quality of food and how it affects the body, which, as I've said, may be key factors in long-term weight regulation.

Laina's Journey

Laina's obsession with calories began when she was a kid. A competitive swimmer growing up, she recalls being weighed in front of the entire team at age 11 to determine her bathing suit

size. Laina had already hit puberty, and though she wasn't over-weight, she felt bigger than everyone else on the team. Seek-ing a solution in one of her mother's diet books, she discovered counting calories. Soon Laina was reading nutrition labels and restricting her food intake to 1,200 calories a day.

As captain of the swim team in high school, she was even more concerned about her appearance, so she obsessively tracked how many calories she burned in her workouts and how many were in everything she put in her mouth, including chewing gum.

When she gained weight in college, Laina returned to calo-rie counting. A pattern developed: She would lose weight, stop tracking calories, and then quickly regain it—plus 10 pounds. She joined online communities of people who shared her preoc-cupation with calories.

In her 20s, Laina went on a supervised, low-calorie shake regimen. She lost 60 pounds in three and a half months but after going back to solid food gained 85 pounds within six months. Blaming herself, Laina thought "I'm a horrible person" because she couldn't manage her weight.

Before long, she was counting calories again, though now she allowed herself 1,500 a day instead of her previous limits of 900 or 1,200. Still, the fixation on calories dominated her life. If invited to a wedding or other social occasion, Laina some-times opted out. "If there was going to be cake," she says, "I just couldn't handle it." When invited out to dinner, she would check the menu ahead of time for a low-calorie option. If she didn't see one, she would make up an excuse not to go.

After Laina moved to Los Angeles for a new job, her weight bumped up again as it had during other transitions in her life. With her wedding coming up, she went on another medically supervised all-shake diet, this time consisting of only 750 calo-ries a day. She lost 50 pounds in time for the big event but then gained 70 over the next two years, reaching her heaviest weight.

Recognizing the toll that all the years of calorie restriction and weight cycling had taken on her physically and mentally, Laina decided to try something new: intuitive eating, which involves listening to the body's hunger cues.

Working with a nutritional therapist, she's learning to think about food in ways that don't involve calories. As a result, she's making healthier choices. For example, after avoiding avocados because of their high calorie count, she says she now views them as "rich in good fat and other great nutrients that your body needs."

Her new outlook is a work in progress. "Whenever I see a piece of food," she says, "in my head I still see a little green number over it with its calorie count." But as she works to liberate herself from that mindset, Laina has developed a healthier relationship with food. She's also healthier physically and emotionally, and at age 38, finally feels she's able to live life fully. "I'm willing to go do things that I wouldn't do before," she says. "It's night and day."

Outmoded Metric

Skeptics of calorie counting often argue that excess calories don't cause obesity and that carbohydrates, fructose, or something else is really responsible. That's not what I'm saying. As discussed in the previous chapter, the case remains unproven that villains such as these are mainly to blame for obesity.

The truth is that calories matter, and you should not ignore them. They're one factor to consider among several—including the nutritional makeup of a food, how it makes you feel, and how much it fills you up—when you're choosing what to eat. But calories shouldn't be the only consideration or necessarily the most important one.

Counting calories can be effective for weight loss in the short term, and it may work long term for some. But for the vast majority of people, it eventually not only fails but also can do harm. For starters, it can detract from the pleasure of eating, turning meals into a tedious exercise of tallying and food weighing. This routine can be stressful and may contribute to an unhealthy relationship with food that makes it even harder to achieve and maintain a healthy weight.

What's more, calorie obsession can lead to food choices and eating habits that undermine your health. Not all calories are the same—50 calories of broccoli doesn't equal 50 calories of jelly beans—and a low-calorie diet is not necessarily a healthy one. Focusing only on calories can result in too little of things your body needs and too much of things it doesn't need.

To say our bodies' weight-regulation mechanisms are complex is an understatement. After many decades of research, there's still much that scientists don't understand and are continuing to discover. So it defies logic that a simple food-scoring system conceived in the 19th century should be adequate for capturing this complexity. Yet calorie counting and calorie math continue to be mainstays of weight-loss efforts.

It is not surprising that our society's preoccupation with this inadequate and error-prone metric has yielded such poor results. What *is* surprising is that we nevertheless continue to give it so much weight.

What to Do

⮑ It's okay to count calories if it works for you. But if not, you don't need to force yourself to do so. Just keep an eye generally on calories in foods.

⮑ When choosing what to eat, also pay attention to other numbers such as the amount of added sugar (the less, the better), fiber (the more, the better), and protein (more can help fill you up). Consider how healthful and filling the foods are, and how you feel after you eat them.

➲ Aim to nourish your body with healthy foods that satisfy your hunger—not to starve yourself.

Chapter 3

EXERCISE ILLUSIONS

I need oxygen," Dom gasped.

"I just gave birth 15 months ago, and I'm in more pain today," said Kristi.

Delores became dizzy.

Phi sobbed.

Kyle vomited. So did Katarina.

So what was causing all this suffering? A war? A terrible illness? A dangerous drug?

Nope, none of the above. It was the weight-loss regimen on TV's *The Biggest Loser*—specifically the exercise routine that participants were subjected to on the first day of the competition.

Like unwanted weight, the popular show went away for a while but then came roaring back. The aforementioned scene was from the new and supposedly improved version, which claimed to put more emphasis on wellness. What didn't change, however, was the show's message that exercise is just as crucial as diet for weight loss.

Or even more so. An analysis of 66 episodes of the original version found that of the time devoted to weight management, 85 percent focused on exercise—more than five times the amount related to diet. What this suggested to viewers, wrote the authors of the analysis, is that "weight loss is achieved primarily through physical activity."

It's not just *The Biggest Loser* that emphasizes the importance of exercise for shedding pounds. So does conventional weight-loss advice based on the calories-in/calories-out model, which is sometimes expressed as ELMM—eat less, move more. ELMM implies that eating and exercise are of equal value for losing weight and that if you fall short on the "eat less" part, you can make up for it by boosting your exercise.

In fact, ELMM Street is a dead end.

The unfortunate truth is that exercise's impact on weight loss is often small to nil. That's because shedding pounds requires more vigorous and sustained activity than most of us are willing or able to do. Plus, as we've seen with diet, the body has ways of resisting our efforts and countering any potential impact that exercise may have on weight.

Nevertheless, many of us cling to the belief that going for a stroll around the block or taking a Pilates class will work off that pepperoni pizza we ate last night and melt away pounds. A US government survey showed just how widespread this view is. Asked to name ways they had tried to slim down, respondents most often mentioned exercise along with eating less. Lagging far behind was "changed eating habits," even though it's a much more effective strategy than exercise.

People who know me find it surprising when I say this because I'm a big proponent of physical activity and an avid exerciser myself. I've even written a book on the subject. There's no question that exercise is essential for good health, providing a wide array of potential benefits from improving your mood to warding off cancer. It may also help *prevent* weight gain and reduce many of the health risks associated with being overweight. So yes, I strongly encourage everyone of all sizes to exercise!

But it's unrealistic to count on exercise to produce weight loss, and doing so can keep people from enjoying the many benefits of physical activity by causing them to become discouraged and give up when it doesn't deliver as promised. In addition, the impression given by *The Biggest Loser* that grueling, push-till-you-puke workouts are necessary to shed pounds may scare many of us off from even trying to lose weight—or exercise. Personally, I know that I would say "no, thanks" to both if I thought they required enduring the hell that those contestants go through.

Of course, playing up exercise makes for good TV. But in reality it's bad advice for weight loss.

Yo-Yo Reasoning

While the idea that exercise promotes weight loss may seem like time-honored wisdom, it actually didn't gain wide acceptance until about 50 years ago. Before then there were hints of it, though.

As early as the 1920s, popular women's magazines portrayed certain exercises as a way to shape readers' bodies. Without mentioning calories burned or pounds shed, articles such as "Stretch and Grow Slim," "Ten Minutes a Day Keep the Bulges Away," and "Six Easy Exercises for the Bosom" advised women to do stretches and other moves targeting specific areas in order to improve their figures and maintain a youthful appearance. The exercises were usually gentle, since strenuous activity was thought to be harmful for women's bodies. And heaven forbid that women should perspire; it was unladylike.

These notions were behind a chain of women's salons called Slenderella, which sprang up in the 1950s. There, clients would lie on vibrating tables, a form of passive exercise that was advertised to "firm and tone" and make women "the size you ought to be." Similarly, vibrating belts, which became iconic "exercise" machines of the 1950s, were a popular way for women to supposedly jiggle away unwanted fat.

Many physicians warned that exercise was unnecessary and even dangerous for middle-aged and older men as well as women. Among the most outspoken exercise skeptics was Dr. Peter Steincrohn, who authored a book in the 1940s titled *You Don't Have to Exercise!*

Steincrohn and others argued that exercise not only wasted energy but also burned too few calories to be effective for weight loss.

Enter Jean Mayer, a nutrition researcher at Harvard who would later become president of Tufts University. Beginning in the 1950s, Mayer was a leading proponent of exercise who, unlike other early fitness evangelists such as Jack LaLanne, had strong scientific credentials. Citing his own research in rodents and people, Mayer championed the idea that a sedentary lifestyle was a major cause of obesity and that physical activity could help curb excess weight. He frequently used popular media to spread the word. For example, writing in the *New York Times* in 1965 under the headline "The Best Diet Is Exercise," Mayer informed readers that a daily game of squash could lead to a loss of 16 pounds over the course of a year.

By the end of the 1960s, Mayer's message that exercise was effective for weight loss had sunk in with the public. During the next several decades, the idea became further entrenched thanks to fitness gurus ranging from Jane Fonda to Richard Simmons to Jillian Michaels. Gyms and personal trainers held out the promise of weight loss as a way to attract clients. Michelle Obama's "Let's Move" campaign pushed physical activity as key to ending childhood obesity. Even Coca-Cola jumped on the bandwagon, funding research as well as a group called the Global Energy Balance Network to promote the importance of "maintaining an active lifestyle" (as opposed to skipping sugary beverages) to combat obesity.

Eventually negative publicity killed Coca-Cola's efforts, but the viewpoint espoused by the company and others—that exercise is an antidote to overeating—refuses to die.

Low ROI

In fact, even if it's vigorous, exercise accounts for a relatively small portion of the calories that we burn each day. The vast majority—two-thirds or more—go toward just keeping the body functioning. As mentioned in the previous chapter, this is known as the basal metabolic rate (BMR) and includes things like breathing, blood circulation, and brain function. Another 10 percent of calories go toward digesting food.

That leaves roughly 25 percent for physical activity, of which there are two types. First are routine activities—everything from brushing your teeth and typing on your laptop to standing, walking around, and even fidgeting. The energy expended on such activities, known as non-exercise activity thermogenesis, or NEAT, varies widely from person to person depending on factors such as occupation (construction workers burn more calories than office workers); age (younger people typically move more than older folks); and season (people tend to be more active in warmer weather).

This brings us to the second type of activity, exercise. How many calories you burn while doing a particular exercise depends on, among other things, your age, weight, gender, and fitness level, as well as how vigorously and for how long you perform the activity.

Take walking, for example. A 150-pound person who walks briskly for 30 minutes will burn around 140 calories. (Again, there are a number of variables, so this is just an estimate.) If you consume, say, 2,000 calories a day, that walk will work off only about 7 percent of those calories. Put another way, that's equal to the calories in one can of Coke—not exactly a great return on your investment of time and effort.

Riding a stationary bike at a moderate pace for 30 minutes, the same person will get a greater yield—250 calories, which is the amount in one standard-size Snickers bar. Step it up to a 10-minute mile run, and they'll burn 350 calories—roughly the number in a Starbucks chocolate chip cookie.

You get the idea: It takes a lot of work to burn off the calories in a relatively small amount of food. Simply skipping the Coke, candy bar, or cookie is far easier.

This helps explain why studies overall show that doing moderate-intensity aerobic exercise such as walking for 30 minutes a day, five days a week—the amount recommended for good health—typically produces little or no weight loss by itself.

When moderate exercise is added to diet, the results are equally unimpressive. Pooling data from six trials, researchers found that a combination of diet and exercise generated no greater weight loss than diet alone after six months. At 12 months, the diet-and-exercise combo showed an advantage, but it was slight—about 4 pounds on average. In another review of studies, the difference was less than 3 pounds.

In studies where exercise *has* produced meaningful weight loss, participants burned at least 400 to 500 calories per session on five or more days a week. To achieve that, a 150-pound person would need to log a minimum of 90 minutes per day of brisk walking or 30 minutes of running eight-minute miles. In short, exercise sessions need to be lengthy or vigorous or both.

High-intensity regimens may also promote weight loss by increasing the number of calories burned *after* the workout.

For up to 24 hours following vigorous exercise, your metabolism can stay revved up, a phenomenon known as excess postexercise oxygen consumption, or EPOC. Also called afterburn, it's basically a calorie-burning bonus while the body recovers.

Though EPOC is typically modest, in some cases the increase can be meaningful. In one small study, for example, young men did 45 minutes of strenuous cycling, burning just over 500 calories on average. During 14 hours after the exercise session, their bodies used an additional 190 calories compared to what they burned on a day with no exercise—a 37 percent boost. Some of this extra calorie burning even occurred while the subjects slept.

High-intensity interval training, or HIIT, which involves alternating short spurts of hard effort with periods of light effort, may be especially effective at raising EPOC, according to some research. But if your regimen consists of something less intense, like 30 minutes of walking, you're unlikely to generate much if any afterburn.

In a way, it's a story of the rich getting richer: Those able to run marathons or do strenuous spin classes burn sufficient calories for weight loss while they exercise—and then torch even more while they rest. Those who can't or won't exercise this vigorously—which is to say the vast majority of us—usually derive neither benefit.

MYTH OR TRUTH?

High-sweat workouts burn more calories.

When body temperature rises, glands in our skin secrete sweat, and the evaporation of this moisture helps cool us off. But how much we sweat doesn't necessarily correlate with how intense a workout is or how many calories we burn. Instead, perspiration depends on a number of factors, including gender (men tend to sweat more than women), age (younger people sweat more than older people), and genetics, as well as the temperature and humidity of our environment. Weight plays a role as well. Larger people tend to perspire more because their bodies generate more heat. Fitness level matters too. Surprisingly, fit people may sweat sooner and more heavily during exercise because their bodies' cooling systems are more efficient, allowing them to work harder.

Heavy sweating can lead to the loss of a few pounds, but this is water weight that's gained back when you rehydrate and isn't necessarily a sign that you've burned lots of calories. On the other hand, a low-sweat workout doesn't necessarily mean low calorie burning. A better indicator is the so-called talk test. If you can talk and sing during your activity without becoming breathless, the intensity level is low. If you can talk but *not* sing, the intensity is moderate. And if you can barely get out any words, you're doing vigorous exercise—and burning more calories.

Exercisers' Compensation

Even if you're one of those people who work their tails off at the gym, there's no guarantee you'll lose a lot of weight— or any at all. The effects of exercise, like diet, vary from person to person—a fact demonstrated by a study in which overweight subjects did supervised high-intensity exercise (burning 500 calories per session) five times a week. After 12 weeks, they shed an average of about 8 pounds. But individual results were all over the map. Some participants lost as much as 20 to 30 pounds while others *gained* a few.

So what explains these differences? One possibility is that vigorous exercise can ramp up appetite, prompting some people to eat more. In that study with wide-ranging results, the researchers fed meals to participants at the beginning and end of the experiment, recording how much they ate. Subjects who had lost less weight than expected (or gained weight) boosted their calorie intake, while the "bigger losers"—those who lost as much as expected or more—did not.

Increased appetite after exercise is an example of what scientists call a *compensatory* response. That is, we compensate for the extra calories burned by eating more in order to maintain energy balance and our weight. This response helped keep our prey-chasing prehistoric ancestors alive, but it can be a problem when we're trying to slim down.

The impulse to eat in response to exercise can be biological as well as psychological. In one study, exercisers who lost less weight than expected reported greater hunger and more cravings for sweets than the more successful losers. The less successful losers were also more likely to believe that "good" health behaviors could counteract "bad" ones— that exercise gave them license to have extra scoops of ice cream, for example.

Such a belief can really lead to trouble when people don't have a firm grasp of how many calories they're burning or eating, which, as discussed in the previous chapter, is often the case. In one experiment, subjects worked out on a treadmill and then estimated how many calories they had burned. They overshot by as much as fourfold on average. Later, when they were taken to a buffet and told to eat the number of calories they had expended through exercise, the participants overestimated again, consuming more than twice as many calories as they had actually burned. The study makes it clear how the attitude "I exercise so I can eat"—something I hear all the time—can be counterproductive and actually lead to weight *gain*.

While increased eating is the most widely recognized form of compensation, it's not the only one. We may also move less after we finish exercising. Though evidence for this idea is mixed, some research does suggest that people who lose less weight than expected from exercise show reductions in NEAT (energy expended on non-exercise activity). They may spend more time sitting in front of the TV, for instance, or less time playing with their kids or doing chores.

One possible reason is that they're fatigued from the exercise. Or perhaps they feel entitled to take it easy because they worked out. Or maybe their bodies compensate with subtle changes like reduced fidgeting, of which they're unaware.

Compensation can also come in the form of a reduced BMR. While vigorous exercise may temporarily boost metabolism, over time it can dial metabolism down. As we become lighter, the body needs less energy to function, so it burns fewer calories. As discussed in chapter 2, losing weight by cutting calories can push BMR lower than it would be for someone of our smaller size who had not dropped pounds. The same thing can happen if we lose weight through exercise.

In a study of overweight and obese women who did vigorous exercise five days a week for three months, almost half experienced greater-than-expected decreases in BMR. These individuals also shed fewer pounds, on average, than the other participants, a result suggesting that variability in BMR changes may be another reason why some people benefit less than others from all their hard work at the gym.

Because of these compensatory responses, we typically have to keep ratcheting up the amount of exercise in order to burn enough calories to continue losing weight. But eventually our bodies stop cooperating. Once we reach a certain exercise threshold, research suggests that total energy expenditure may plateau so that running more or spinning harder ceases to result in any additional calorie burning. The extra effort, in other words, stops paying off for weight loss.

The science is sparse on whether genetics plays a role in compensatory responses, and if so, which genes are responsible. But it's certainly plausible that genetic differences help explain why vigorous exercise causes some people to lose more weight than others. After all, we know that cardiovascular fitness levels vary greatly in response to aerobic exercise, for example. Some people experience big improvements, while others see little or no change. By one estimate, as much as half of this variation is due to heredity. So it stands to reason that our weight-related responses to exercise likewise depend at least partly on our genetic makeup.

Whatever the case, this much is certain: The advice to "move more" in order to weigh less fails to account for the complexity of how our bodies actually work. Like other bromides, this one should be swallowed with an abundance of caution.

MYTH OR TRUTH?

Calorie counts on cardio machines and fitness trackers are accurate.

Some cardio machines allow users to enter their weight and age, which helps improve accuracy. (Heavier people burn more calories from a given activity, as do those who are younger.) But the machines don't take into account other factors that can affect energy expenditure, including:

➲ **Body fat:** People with less fat and more muscle mass burn more calories.

⊃ **Fitness level:** Beginners burn more calories because they're less efficient at the activity.

⊃ **Form:** Treadmill users who hold on to the handrails, for example, burn fewer calories.

As a result, calorie counts can be off by as much as 20 percent or more. Elliptical machines are especially prone to overestimating calorie burn, while stationary bikes tend to be the most accurate.

Calorie readings on wearable fitness trackers are also often unreliable. In a study of seven devices, the most accurate was off by 27 percent; the least accurate missed the mark by more than 90 percent. Still, calorie counts from machines and devices aren't entirely useless. They can help you gauge the intensity of your workout and indicate whether it's increasing for a particular activity from one day to another.

Warding Off Weight Gain

Though exercise is typically an ineffective way to lose weight, it may help with an even bigger challenge: preventing lost weight from returning.

Consider the experience of participants in the National Weight Control Registry, which studies those who have lost at least 30 pounds and kept it off long term. More than 85 percent report doing physical activity on a regular basis, with about half getting in an hour or more a day.

Likewise, a study involving overweight women found that those who managed to keep off at least 10 percent of their initial body weight for two years exercised an average of about an hour a day, five days a week. Participants who did less exercise regained more weight.

Further evidence comes from research involving 14 contestants on *The Biggest Loser*. After initially shedding about

130 pounds on average, most of the participants regained a significant amount of weight over the next six years. How much depended on how much exercise they were doing. Those who were more successful at keeping weight off tended to be quite active—though at levels below the vomit-inducing intensity from the early weeks of the competition.

Exercise can also help stave off weight gain in the first place. A study that followed participants for 20 years found that the most active men put on an average of 6 fewer pounds than their couch-potato peers as they moved from young adulthood into middle age. Active women experienced an even greater benefit, gaining 13 fewer pounds than inactive women. Researchers controlled for other factors such as calorie consumption that might explain the findings. Similarly, a study that gathered data on 19,000 Norwegians over the course of more than 20 years found that physically active adults of all ages, including those over 60, gained less weight than those who were inactive.

Nevertheless, exercise doesn't completely ward off weight gain. In the Norwegian study, the physically active participants still tended to put on at least some weight over time. It's also worth noting that this study, like much of the other research on the topic of exercise and weight-gain prevention, is observational, so it doesn't prove cause and effect. But taken together, the studies provide strong circumstantial evidence that exercise can in fact limit weight gain, whether initially or after weight loss.

As for how much activity is optimal, the findings conflict, and individuals' results often vary. Some people who keep extra pounds at bay do a lot of exercise, while others do moderate or lighter amounts. Overall, however, research suggests that levels of at least 150 minutes a week (the amount recommended for good health) are effective and that more is better.

MYTH OR TRUTH?

Aerobic exercise is the most effective type for weight control.

Aerobic (or cardio) exercises such as brisk walking, running, and cycling—whether done continuously or in intervals as part of a HIIT workout—typically burn more calories than resistance exercises such as weight lifting, so aerobic activities generally have a greater effect on weight. However, like cardio, resistance training can decrease body fat even if you don't lose weight. In addition, resistance exercises may help you maintain or gain muscle mass, something that's especially important if you're on a low-calorie diet, which can cause the loss of muscle. It's also true that having more muscle mass may result in greater calorie expenditure, since a pound of muscle burns more calories than a pound of fat. But the difference is relatively small, and most of us aren't able to add enough muscle through resistance training to have a meaningful effect on calorie burning. Still, for both weight control and overall health, the best approach is to incorporate both aerobic and resistance exercises.

Fit vs. Fat

If you exercise regularly, you may find that your clothes are looser around your waist even though the scale doesn't show you've lost an ounce. So how can this be? Exercise can reduce visceral fat, the type that's deep in the abdomen and surrounds the liver and other internal organs. Though we can't see visceral fat—it's different from so-called subcutaneous fat, which you can pinch—a large waist is usually a sign of excess visceral fat. (For more on waist size and visceral fat, see chapter 7.)

Combining data from more than 100 studies, researchers found that exercise was less effective for weight loss than calorie-restricted diets. No surprise there. But here's the interesting part: Exercise was *more* effective at reducing visceral fat. In people who didn't lose any weight, exercise resulted in a 6 percent decrease in visceral fat, while diet led to virtually no change.

The upshot is that exercise can shrink your waist and make you look slimmer, even if it doesn't lead to weight loss. (I should note here that "exercise" means aerobic activities, resistance training, or some combination—but not hundreds of crunches. Contrary to popular belief, abdominal exercises can't banish belly fat.)

This benefit isn't just cosmetic. Visceral fat is thought to wreak havoc in the body by producing inflammation-causing compounds and releasing fatty acids into the liver—effects that may help explain why higher amounts of visceral fat go hand in hand with an increased risk of heart disease, diabetes, and premature death. By reducing this type of fat, exercise can help improve your health regardless of your weight.

Exercise can also affect the body in other ways—from improving circulation to controlling blood sugar—that may be especially beneficial for people who are heavy and consequently face greater health risks.

How big a dent exercise makes has been debated for decades. Some research suggests that exercise can completely eliminate certain negative health effects linked to obesity. For example, pooling data from 10 studies, researchers found that heavier people who are fit have no higher risk of premature death than lean, fit people. There's also evidence that those who are fat but fit actually tend to live *longer* than lean couch potatoes.

However, other research has not shown that fitness matters more than fatness. In one study, for instance, the odds of developing risk factors for heart disease such as high blood pressure and abnormal cholesterol rose as people gained body fat. If over time they also became more fit (as measured by treadmill tests), their risk was still elevated, though less so.

Whichever studies you choose, here's what they agree on: Exercise can reduce—perhaps greatly—many of the health risks associated with excess weight. And you don't have to do a huge amount. Getting at least 30 minutes a day of physical activity—which you can accumulate in shorter increments—five days a week can do the trick. You may not lose weight, but you stand to gain something even more valuable: better health.

Kristy's Journey

As a competitive dancer in high school, Kristy was always aware of her body size and focused on burning enough calories to have the right "look" and fit into her costumes. When she got to college, she stopped competing and exercising. "I was so done with it," she says, after having spent so much time in the dance studio.

During college and the years afterward, she put on weight. But whenever a wedding or other special event was coming up, Kristy would diet and exercise to look good in the clothes she wanted to wear. She disliked the workouts but saw them as a necessary evil to reach her goal. Once the special occasion was over, she'd return to her previous lifestyle. Within months, she would regain the weight she had lost—sometimes as much as 30 pounds—and then some.

Throughout her 20s and 30s, the yo-yo dieting continued, with each cycle resulting in a higher weight. Approaching her 40th birthday, Kristy struggled to climb stairs with a load of laundry and was on medication for high blood pressure. She felt physically and emotionally exhausted. "I was tired of being tired," she says. "I knew my body could do more."

So she decided to try physical activity for a week to see if it could help. Dusting off an old series of exercise videos, she found it tough to get through the routine on the first day. But she tried again the next day. And the next. By the end of the first week, Kristy could make it through the 20-minute workout without stopping. Instead of getting on a scale, she focused on how she felt, noting how her breathing, sleep quality, and mood had all improved.

That motivated her to keep going. From there, she increased her amount of daily exercise in small increments, keeping her goals achievable. Not one for gyms or group classes, she found other DVDs and YouTube videos to incorporate cardio, strength training, and Pilates-style exercises for flexibility. She treated her workouts as appointments that she couldn't cancel.

Kristy applied the same healthy lifestyle approach to eating, setting small, measurable goals and not beating herself up for splurging. She made a point never to use exercise as a way to eat more or compensate for overindulging, as she had in the past. "I'm not exercising to eat," she says. "I'm exercising to be healthier."

Today, she works out every day, even when she travels, and looks forward to it. "Exercise is not the enemy anymore," she says. "It's not a punishment."

Thanks to her healthier lifestyle, Kristy no longer needs blood pressure medicine. Her weight is down by more than 100 pounds, though her main focus isn't the scale. What matters most, she says, is how great she feels, both physically and mentally.

Unreasonable Demands

Imagine a pill that could lower your risk of heart disease, stroke, cancer, diabetes, dementia, depression, colds, back pain, osteoporosis, and premature death. It could also improve sleep, boost energy, reduce anxiety, fend off old-age feebleness, and even enhance our sex lives. We'd all be clamoring for it!

Exercise can do all those things and more. Yet our main expectation for exercise is often one of the few things it usually can't do: melt away pounds. Talk about demanding too much.

The weight-loss industry has taken what should be a way to enhance the quality of our lives and turned it into something that we *must* do to shed pounds. In the process, exercise has been set up to fail. And so have we by being conditioned to think of working out as the price we have to pay for a slimmer body.

Sometimes we view this price as penance for overindulging. How many times have you heard someone say—or said yourself—"I'll need to do extra exercise" after eating too much during the holidays or at a celebratory dinner? We treat exercise as a form of self-punishment for being "bad."

When exercise fails to meet our unrealistic expectations, we often sour on it and stop working out. In a study of 30 overweight people who participated in a 12-week exercise program and were interviewed afterward, this response was typical: "It was quite disappointing that I didn't lose a single pound and . . . it kind of made me give up, and I went back to my old routine." Another respondent who failed to lose weight described her exercise experience as "like banging my head against a brick wall." It's pretty safe to assume she didn't go back for more.

In another study, researchers asked middle-aged women to write down their thoughts about physical activity. Those who used terms like "calories" or "weight" were labeled "body-shapers," while those who didn't were called "non-body-shapers." Both groups weighed about the same on average. The body-shapers were more likely to view exercise as a struggle, while the non-body-shapers tended to say that it made them feel good. Given such attitudes, it's not surprising that the body-shapers exercised considerably less than the non-body-shapers.

The takeaway from this research is that we're more likely to perceive exercise positively and actually do it when we focus on our well-being rather than our weight. For some, the incentive may be an improved mood or less stress. Others may find that exercise makes them feel physically and mentally stronger or more in control of their lives. Still others may be motivated by better heart health.

Emphasizing such benefits can actually enhance our weight-control efforts. When we see exercise as something that we *want* to do for ourselves instead of something we *have* to do for our weight, we may be less likely to reward our efforts with food. The payoff comes from how exercise makes us feel—what psychologists call "intrinsic" motivation—so there's less need for a postworkout prize in the form of a Frappuccino or frozen yogurt.

Our relationship with food may benefit in other ways, too. When we use exercise to help us feel better physically and psychologically, we may be more inclined to make healthy, weight-friendly food choices. And because we feel more empowered and less stressed, we may be better able to resist emotional eating.

In addition, decoupling exercise from weight control may improve our odds of avoiding weight gain. I know this sounds contradictory, but here's why it's not: As discussed previously, exercise can help keep added weight at bay—but only if we stick with it long term. Weight-driven exercise is often a short-term endeavor. We stop once we reach a goal or give up in frustration when we don't. Or we push ourselves to the max to burn lots of calories, and as with extreme diets, we eventually abandon the regimen. When we exercise for reasons other than weight management, we're more likely to continue for the long haul.

In the ways I describe above, framing exercise as a weight-loss tool has ironically diminished its potential to control our weight. And, worse than that, this misguided effort has kept us from fully enjoying the health- and life-enhancing benefits of moving our bodies. Weight-loss gurus, fitness advocates, doctors, health officials, health clubs, and others who encourage us to exercise to lose weight may be motivated by the best of intentions. But their advice has caused harm by diverting our efforts away from more effective weight-loss approaches and inadvertently making us less likely to exercise. We'd be far better off if they told us the truth: that we should focus on movement for its own sake—and forget about how it moves the needle on the scale.

What to Do

- ⮑ Try to get in at least 30 minutes a day, five days a week, of aerobic activities that you enjoy. It's fine to break the time into smaller chunks. In addition, do resistance exercises at least twice a week.

- ⮑ Don't expect exercise to melt away pounds, and don't use it to compensate for overeating. Instead, view exercise as a way to enhance your well-being. Focus on its short-term benefits such as better sleep, less stress, or a feeling of empowerment.

- ⮑ To stay motivated, team up with a friend or join a class. Schedule exercise at a time when you're most likely to do it, and make it a priority. Choose a convenient place to work out where you feel comfortable; it doesn't have to be a gym.

Chapter 4

SUPERFOOD FOOLERY

If I had to name things I couldn't live without, chocolate would be high on the list. Whether it's candy, ice cream, cookies, or brownies, I have a hard time resisting anything that contains chocolate. To satisfy my craving, I eat a little chocolate (okay, sometimes more than a little) virtually every day.

Maybe I was an Aztec in a previous life. Like me, the Aztecs loved chocolate. In fact, they considered it a gift from the gods, believing that it conferred wisdom, boosted sex drive, and enhanced warriors' prowess. They even used cacao beans, from which chocolate is made, as money and regarded them as more valuable than gold.

Throughout history, other cultures have also attributed magical powers to certain foods. For example, women in ancient Rome wore cucumbers around their waists to boost fertility. Ancient Egyptians thought that onions could revive the dead as they journeyed to the afterlife. In ancient Greece, Olympic athletes consumed garlic to give them an edge in competition. And emperors in ancient China ate black rice (commoners weren't allowed to have it) to ensure a long and healthy life.

Today we have our own versions of magical foods. We call them superfoods—specific foods containing substances ranging from alpha-linolenic acid to zeaxanthin that allegedly have the power to ward off illness and keep us healthy.

Do a quick Internet search for superfoods, and here's a small sampling of what you'll find: Prunes boost bone density. Blueberries improve memory. Cauliflower prevents cancer. Kiwis fight asthma. Sweet potatoes enhance vision. Bok choy makes your skin glow. Pomegranates increase testosterone. Chia seeds strengthen immunity.

And of course I can't forget chocolate: The dark version is supposedly good for both your heart and your brain. (The Aztecs would undoubtedly approve.)

When it comes to superfoods for weight loss, perhaps the most iconic is grapefruit. For decades, the fruit has been touted as a ticket to a slimmer body. In the 1930s, it was the star attraction of the Hollywood diet (also known as the 18-Day diet), a very low-calorie regimen that involved eating a grapefruit at every meal.

Since then, the grapefruit diet has reappeared in different forms. Today grapefruit juice and even grapefruit capsules have been incorporated into the diet and a new rationale added: that grapefruit contains special fat-burning enzymes. In fact, there's no evidence for the claim. While grapefruit, like other fruits, can help with weight control by filling you up, there's nothing uniquely beneficial about it.

The same goes for most other superfoods. They often belong to broad categories such as vegetables, fruits, legumes, nuts, and fish, which research shows to be part of a healthy and weight-friendly diet. But the notion that specific foods, in isolation, have the power to peel away pounds is scientifically baseless.

That hasn't stopped the news media, food manufacturers, social media influencers, and even doctors from hyping the superpowers of certain foods for weight loss. Often they do so by exaggerating preliminary research—much of it funded by vested interests—and making it seem far more definitive or relevant than it actually is.

Duped by this scientific distortion, we end up buying and eating more of particular foods—an outcome that expands food producers' bottom lines but doesn't shrink our waistlines.

The list of these foods is so long that reviewing them all could fill an entire book, so I won't even try. Instead, I'll focus here on a few of the most common ones, which help illustrate where messages about fat-zapping foods come from and how they're misleading.

Bitter Truth

One of the most ballyhooed superfoods for weight loss these days is apple cider vinegar, or ACV for short. The stuff has a strong, bitter taste that most people find pretty awful, a fact that makes ACV's growing popularity in recent years especially remarkable.

Among those most responsible for its salubrious status is Dr. Mehmet Oz, whose popular TV show has repeatedly beaten the drum for ACV's alleged benefits. Dr. Oz's "swim-suit slim-down plan" includes swallowing two tablespoons of ACV (mixed with grapefruit juice) before every meal. By doing so, he claims, "you'll literally burn away your fat."

The Kardashians are big ACV boosters as well. Kourtney drinks a tablespoon twice a day, which is supposedly one of the keys to her impressive body. Khloé reportedly consumes ACV three times a day in order to rev up her metabolism. And Kim has plugged a book about ACV, titled *Apple Cider Vinegar: Miracle Health System*, to her 200-plus million followers on Instagram.

The book—authored by Patricia Bragg and the late Paul Bragg, whose names and faces adorn their brand of ACV—proclaims on the cover that ACV can "control weight and banish obesity." A section titled "ACV Miracle for Overweight" explains that the "acidic nature of ACV helps stimulate [a] bodily response that burns stored fat that accelerates weight loss!"

Indeed there is some evidence that acetic acid, the main component of ACV and other vinegars, affects genes involved in the formation and breakdown of fat, and reduces body weight and fat accumulation. But what ACV proponents often neglect to mention is that this research was done on rodents, a fact that limits its relevance unless you're a fat rat.

As for research in people, the most frequently cited study involved 155 overweight participants who were assigned to consume a beverage that contained either zero, 1, or 2 tablespoons of apple cider vinegar daily. After 12 weeks, those taking ACV lost weight. But the amount was relatively small—just 2 to 4 pounds. And notably, the study was conducted by a Japanese food company that sells vinegar.

From there, the evidence gets weaker. A few small studies show that vinegar may reduce spikes in blood sugar after meals. While some theorize that this can lead to weight loss, it remains unproven. There's also research suggesting that vinegar may decrease appetite—but at least one study found that's because the vinegar made subjects nauseated. Hardly an ideal way to control eating!

Nausea isn't the only potential negative effect of ACV. If not sufficiently diluted, it can eat away tooth enamel and damage the esophagus.

ACV pills and gummies are touted as a way to avoid these effects, along with the strong taste. But these products, like other dietary supplements, are only loosely regulated, so we can't be sure whether they're safe or even what they contain. (For more on weight-loss supplements, see chapter 6.)

Consumerlab.com, an independent organization that tests supplements, has found that the concentration of acetic acid in ACV pills varies widely, from as little as 0.4 percent to more than 30 percent. As the group points out, any product containing more than 20 percent acetic acid is considered a poison by US government safety regulators. So instead of being safer than liquid, some ACV supplements might actually pose a bigger risk.

Even if the risk is low, the fact remains that compelling evidence for ACV is MIA, regardless of whether the vinegar comes in liquid or solid form.

MYTH OR TRUTH?

Drinking lots of water helps you lose weight.

The most common explanation for this widely held belief is that water fills you up and dampens hunger. Indeed there's some evidence that water does have an effect—if you drink at the right time. In studies, drinking 2 cups 30 minutes before meals resulted in greater weight loss—by 3 to 4 pounds over 12 weeks—compared to having no water before meals. The most diligent premeal drinkers shed about 8 pounds more. Interestingly, though, the 30-minute window appears to be effective only for middle-aged and older folks. To reduce hunger, younger people may need to drink immediately before eating, perhaps because water empties more rapidly from their stomachs and they don't stay full as long.

There's no solid evidence, though, that drinking lots of water overall affects weight. Nor, despite the claims, is there proof that "functional" waters like alkaline and oxygenated water have special fat-burning abilities or are superior to regular water for weight loss.

Fat Chance

"Eat more of coconut oil and you might slim your waist size in one week," declares the headline of an article by Dr. Joseph Mercola. Elsewhere on his "natural health" website, which attracts millions of people, Mercola claims that the oil can "stimulate your metabolism, helping you shed body fat." (Never mind that he also happens to sell coconut oil.)

Thanks to such pronouncements by Mercola and others, coconut oil has gained a reputation as a miracle food for weight loss. Its proponents attribute this and other alleged health benefits to a type of fat in coconut oil known as medium-chain triglycerides, or MCTs.

By contrast, other vegetable oils such as soybean and olive consist entirely of fats called long-chain triglycerides (LCTs). Our bodies process MCTs differently than LCTs, a fact thought to explain why MCTs have been shown to increase fullness and rev up metabolism. What's more, trials comparing MCTs with LCTs suggest that MCTs may slightly reduce weight and body fat.

But there's a catch: All this research involves pure MCT oil, which is not the same as coconut oil. While coconut oil has a relatively high percentage of MCTs, the levels are lower than those in MCT oil. And the two oils differ in their exact makeup of fatty acids.

In a way, what we have here is a bait-and-switch. The promises made to us about coconut oil actually apply (sort of) to something else. It's like being sold a car that supposedly has all the latest bells and whistles and can go from 0 to 60 mph in three seconds, only to find out when you take it home that the salesman was describing a different car.

So what do we know about our actual purchase, coconut oil? Not much.

One of the few published studies, conducted by a student in Brazil for a master's degree thesis, involved 40 young women who were instructed to eat a low-calorie diet and walk every day. Half consumed 2 tablespoons of coconut oil daily, while the others took in the same amount of soybean oil. After 12 weeks, the coconut oil eaters, but not the soybean oil group, experienced a slight decrease in waist size. But both groups fared the same when it came to weight loss, dropping about 2 pounds on average.

Other small, short-term studies have also failed to show any effect of coconut oil on weight. Noting the dearth of research, one review of studies concluded that claims about coconut oil and weight are "unrealistic and unsupported by scientific evidence."

On the flip side, there is considerable evidence that the high concentration of saturated fat in coconut oil raises LDL cholesterol, the type linked to an increased risk of heart disease. Though the oil also elevates HDL, the good cholesterol, it's unclear whether this is beneficial for heart health.

So, with coconut oil, we get no proven benefit for weight control and at least the possibility of harm to our hearts. Thanks, but I'll pass on that deal.

MYTH OR TRUTH?

Bulletproof coffee promotes weight loss.

Add 1 to 2 tablespoons each of MCT oil and unsalted butter to a cup of brewed coffee, and you get so-called bulletproof coffee, which celebrities and athletes have embraced as a keto-friendly substitute for breakfast. Developed by Silicon Valley entrepreneur Dave Asprey, the 450-calorie concoction can supposedly control weight by suppressing hunger while also increasing energy and mental sharpness. But there's no published data supporting the claims.

When it comes to regular (i.e., nonbulletproof) coffee, some research suggests that drinking 4 cups a day may modestly reduce body fat, likely because of the caffeine. (For more about the effects of caffeine on weight, see chapter 6.) But if you load up your morning joe with cream and sugar, or your coffee of choice is a Double Chocolaty Chip Frappuccino, I wouldn't count on it.

Another high-fat superfood, avocado, doesn't have the drawbacks of coconut oil. The main type of fat that avocados contain, monounsaturated fat, is thought to be heart healthy. This "good" fat also supposedly helps account for the fruit's purported power to melt away pounds.

It's a message we see repeatedly in news reports. Take, for example, a widely distributed story headlined "Avocados May Be the Key to Weight Loss, Study Says." The lead paragraph informed readers about "a new study . . . that suggests the fat in avocado can help you suppress hunger."

In that study, researchers fed 31 overweight and obese subjects three different breakfasts: a high-fat meal that included one avocado; a high-fat meal with half an avocado; and a low-fat, high-carbohydrate meal that served as a control. All meals contained about the same number of calories. For six hours after each meal, subjects reported how hungry or full they felt.

Notably, there was no measurement of how much they actually ate after the meal or what happened to their weight. But you wouldn't know that from reading the news story, which concluded that "swapping a piece of bread for a yummy half-avocado can help you achieve your weight loss goals."

Really? Based on a six-hour study that didn't track any-one's weight?

There was also this glaring omission: The study was funded by the Hass Avocado Board.

In fact, much of the research on avocados and weight has been sponsored by this industry group, which represents avocado producers and importers. The board supports studies through its nutrition research program, the stated aim of which is "to discover and validate the role of fresh avocados to improve public health." Or, as the board put it when the initiative was announced, the research is intended to "help confirm what many people have known all along—that avocados are a super food."

Essentially, the effort is about using science to generate headlines and market avocados. And it benefits nearly everyone involved: Researchers get funding, which they need to survive professionally. Universities producing the research and academic journals publishing it get attention through press releases they issue. News outlets get stories from these releases about weight-reducing foods, which are guaranteed to attract eyeballs. And the avocado industry gets increased sales of its product.

Conspicuously absent from the list of beneficiaries is the public, which is misled to believe that avocados have magical fat-melting abilities.

To see beyond the spin, we need to look at the evidence as a whole. In the case of avocados and weight, there isn't much, and what we have is far from persuasive. Even a trial sponsored by the Hass Avocado Board found that adding an avocado to a low-calorie diet for 12 weeks resulted in no greater weight loss than the diet alone.

What we do know is that avocados, like nuts and certain other fatty foods, can be part of a healthful diet that helps control weight. So enjoy an avocado or some guacamole if you like the taste. But that should be the reason—not weight-loss hype from industry and the media.

Haley's Journey

Haley grew up in a family where being overweight was the norm. When she began playing sports in middle school, her weight went down. That made her happy, so she started watching what she ate, and more pounds dropped off.

When the weight loss stopped, she began tracking every calorie through an app and turned to extreme exercise. At age 15, she developed anorexia.

In her teens and 20s, Haley tried a number of fad diets. When one stopped working, she moved on to the next. She also latched on to superfoods after seeing fitness enthusiasts rave about them on social media. "So of course I had to go buy 20 servings and eat them immediately," she says.

Haley spent days eating only kale for every meal. She drank apple cider vinegar until it made her sick. Grapefruit became a daily staple even though she hated it. "It didn't matter if I liked it or not," she says. "It was going in my mouth."

She believed that eating these foods would make her healthy while also speeding up her metabolism and burning fat. In addition, as someone obsessed with counting calories, Haley liked that these foods tend to be on the low side. She used them to replace higher-calorie foods and reduce her overall calorie intake, even though the replaced foods often supplied nutrients that she needed for a balanced diet.

Just as she had with diets, Haley went from food to food. Eventually she realized that most of it she didn't like, and as a college student, couldn't afford. Plus, the foods didn't help her lose weight.

Now in her late 20s, Haley has developed a much healthier relationship with food. She no longer tracks calories or replaces meals with kale. Instead, she listens to her body and eats what makes her feel good.

"It's a complete difference from where I was," she says. "So I've come a long way."

Hot Air

Topping many lists of fat-reducing foods are hot peppers, for which you can find lots of spicy promises. According to CBSnews.com, they can "fire up weight loss." *Redbook* claims they "supercharge your metabolism." And *Eat This, Not That!* calls them the "best food on the planet for weight loss."

These purported benefits are typically attributed to capsaicin, the compound that gives peppers their kick. Capsaicin supposedly works its magic by curbing appetite, ramping up metabolism, and burning fat.

Though research overall is mixed, there is some evidence for these effects from animal studies and small, short-term human experiments. In a Danish study, for example, 24 subjects ate a series of buffet-style meals, before which they consumed 0.9 grams (about ½ teaspoon) of red pepper, either in tomato juice or capsules. They ate roughly 10 to 15 percent fewer calories and reported feeling more full after ingesting the pepper compared to a placebo.

In another study, 25 subjects consumed meals both with and without 1 gram of red pepper. Metabolism increased for several hours after the peppery meals. The study, along with others on the subject, was funded by the McCormick Science Institute—the same McCormick whose name graces containers of red pepper and other spices.

This study comes with other caveats as well. Regular eaters of red pepper got less of a metabolism boost than those who didn't eat it at all, a result suggesting that our bodies become desensitized to the effects of peppers, just as our taste buds do. Overall, the impact was small—people burned just 10 extra calories, on average, after consuming pepper. By one estimate, for a middle-aged man, that would add up to a whopping 1-pound weight loss over 6.5 years.

Studies using higher doses of capsaicin, given in capsules, show larger upticks in calorie burning, but typically they're still too small to make a difference. In one of the only studies that actually tracked people's weight, 91 subjects received either capsaicin capsules or a placebo for three months after a weight-loss diet. Though fat burning was a bit higher in the capsaicin group, there was no effect on weight, with both groups regaining the same amount. And the capsaicin dose was so high that some of those taking it complained of burning in their stomachs. (Overdoing it on spicy peppers in food form can similarly lead to stomach pain and other gastrointestinal problems.)

Overall, what the research suggests is that you likely need to consume lots of hot peppers—more than many of us are willing to eat or able to tolerate—to affect appetite and metabolism, and even then, the impact is small and short-lived. Most important, there's no proof that eating peppers actually leads to weight loss.

So, while hot peppers can be great for adding zest to your meals, don't expect them to subtract pounds from your body. And, unfortunately, that spicy salsa won't cancel out the chips that accompany it.

MYTH OR TRUTH?

Certain aromas reduce hunger.

Some reports tout sniffing particular scents ranging from peppermint to ginger as a way to lose weight. These smells supposedly send a message to the brain's appetite control center, telling it we're full. In one of the only published studies testing the idea, overweight subjects shed pounds after inhaling a blend of peppermint, banana, and green apple whenever they were hungry. But because the research lacked a control group, it didn't actually prove that the scents were responsible.

Dr. Alan Hirsch, the study's author and chief cheerleader for the connection between aromas and weight loss, is also the developer of Sensa crystals, a product sprinkled onto foods to enhance their aromas and allegedly promote weight loss. (In 2014, the US Federal Trade Commission charged Hirsch and his company with deceptive advertising and assessed a $26.5 million fine.) While other research suggests that scents may curb cravings, it's far from proven which ones are effective, how long the effects last, and whether they promote weight loss. There's more evidence that certain aromas can stimulate appetite. But most of us already know that from getting a whiff of McDonald's fries or a Cinnabon shop.

Produce Promises

Many foods promoted for weight loss fall under the heading of fruits and vegetables, which health authorities encourage us to eat in abundance not only to prevent chronic diseases but also to control weight. Indeed, observational studies (which show associations but not cause and effect) have linked eating more produce to less weight gain. Fruits and veggies are thought to help with weight *loss* because they tend to be filling and relatively low in calories.

Heeding the message, more people now say they're upping their intake of fruits, vegetables, and salads to slim down. In one survey, this ranked among the most commonly reported weight-loss methods, surpassed only by eating less and exercising.

For this strategy to succeed, though, fruits and vegetables need to be a *substitute* for foods like chips, cookies, and fries. Too often, this caveat isn't clear in headlines such as "Fruits, Vegetables May Be Key to Long-Term Weight Loss" and articles telling us that "adding fruits and vegetables to your diet can provide you with speedy weight loss with results that are much more likely to last."

The implication is that simply adding produce to our diets can help us shed pounds. In essence, fruits and vegetables, as a whole, are misleadingly portrayed as fat-banishing superfoods.

Experimental research reveals how this view can lead us astray. In a Scottish study, 62 adults with relatively low intakes of fruits and vegetables were randomly assigned to receive either 600 grams (1.3 pounds) of produce a day, half that amount daily, or none. Recipients were told to include the fruits and vegetables in their diets but not instructed how to make other changes. And in fact they didn't make any. Over the two-month course of the study, the produce eaters lost no more weight than the controls.

A review of this and other randomized trials concluded there's no evidence that eating more fruits and vegetables, without other changes, leads to weight loss. Another such review, which also included the Scottish study, left open the possibility that simply ramping up fruit and vegetable intake "may" contribute to weight loss. But the apparent benefit was so small as to be virtually meaningless.

How fruits and veggies affect weight also has to do with how they're prepared. Fresh peaches, for example, are not the same as canned peaches in heavy syrup. Steamed broccoli is a far cry from broccoli casserole made with cheese, butter, and a crushed-cracker topping. Eating lots of unhealthy, high-calorie forms of produce such as these won't result in weight loss and could very well lead to weight gain.

So why do we keep seeing the oversimplified message that eating more fruits and veggies will magically melt away pounds, without the caution that it matters what the foods replace and how they're prepared?

One reason is that the advice is easier for us to swallow when dished up that way. We're more likely to heed messages involving simple steps we can take that don't require big changes or sacrifices. And just adding some lettuce, tomatoes, or oranges to whatever we're currently eating is about as simple and sacrifice-free as it gets. While this approach may benefit our health by boosting levels of certain nutrients in our diets, it's unlikely to do anything for our weight.

A similar dynamic applies to the promotion of places where we can buy fruits and vegetables—farmers' markets. Often they're touted as a way not only to improve health but also to combat obesity. A press release for one farmers' market put it this way: "To fight an epidemic of obesity . . . faculty and students at the University of Texas School of Public Health Brownsville Regional Campus have come up with a strong weapon: a farmer's market loaded with fresh fruits and vegetables."

By giving us access to fresh produce, we're told, farmers' markets can help us control our weight. Proponents claim they're especially beneficial for low-income communities with so-called food deserts, where the availability of fresh fruits and vegetables is limited.

Now, before I continue, I should note that I am a big fan of farmers' markets and shop at them regularly. They allow you not only to buy super-fresh, delicious produce, but also to learn firsthand how it's grown, discover new foods, and support local farmers. Plus, it's fun to stroll through a farmers' market on a nice day.

In short, there are many good reasons to visit farmers' markets. But weight control is not one of them.

As discussed, the fruits and veggies you get there won't, by themselves, peel away pounds. What's more, alongside the produce you'll typically find all kinds of other foods that are decidedly not healthy or weight friendly. In a survey of

26 farmers' markets in New York City, one-third of the items were refined or processed foods like cookies, croissants, and jams. At my local farmers' market, the booth with the longest line sells ice cream.

The fact that some of these products, such as juices and zucchini bread, have fruits or vegetables as an ingredient can make them *seem* healthy. The same goes for foods with labels like "fresh," "natural," "gluten-free," or "organic," which are ubiquitous at farmers' markets. As I mentioned in chapter 2, when foods have a "health halo," we're more likely to underestimate their calories and overeat them.

By tempting us with unhealthy foods and giving them a healthy imprimatur, farmers' markets don't deliver on their promise of promoting weight loss and may even have the opposite effect. If you go intending to buy apples and end up coming home with an apple pie as well, and along the way treat yourself to a cinnamon roll or ham-and-cheese empanada, that visit will have done no favors for your waistline.

To be clear, I'm not saying you should avoid farmers' markets. By all means support them. Just stick with fruits, vegetables, and other healthful items. Farmers' markets can indeed be magical—but not necessarily for your weight.

MYTH OR TRUTH?

You should consume a variety of foods.

Eating a varied diet would seem to be the sensible alternative to focusing on specific foods. In fact, it may not be. There's little evidence that this time-honored advice results in better health, and it may be counterproductive when it comes to our weight. Research suggests that greater dietary variety can prompt us to eat more because of a phenomenon known as *sensory-specific satiety*: The more we consume a particular food, the less pleasure we derive from it, and the less motivated we become to eat it. Meanwhile, our appetite for other foods persists and may even grow. This explains why, for example, we can be full from dinner but still have room for dessert. Or why we tend to eat more at buffets: When you've had enough of, say, the roast beef, the quiche may still be calling your name.

In some research, consuming a narrow range of foods is associated with better weight control. But limited variety need not apply to fruits and vegetables. Eating lots of different types may benefit both your weight and your health, and keep your meals from becoming monotonous.

False Heroes

If you think about it, superfoods and banned foods are really two sides of the same coin. Both approaches to weight loss turn specific foods into characters in a professional wrestling match, with some assuming the roles of heroes and others playing villains. And we're in the ring too. If we embrace the good guys who can save us or banish the bad guys who will destroy us, we'll supposedly win the battle against our weight.

Like off-limits foods, the concept of weight-loss superfoods appeals to our desire for simple solutions. All we have to do is gulp down some apple cider vinegar or green tea or hot peppers and then let the heroic foods work their magic.

This promise can be all the more alluring when we hear that there's scientific evidence for the effects of a particular food. But as we've seen, the "proof" typically amounts to a grain of truth mixed with a gallon of exaggeration.

Falling for this hype and fixating on fat-burning foods distracts us from where our focus should be—our overall diets.

And overdoing it on calorically dense superfoods like coconut oil or nuts can potentially backfire and fuel weight gain.

Fairy tales often include a false hero who claims to save the day while thwarting the true hero's efforts. That's basically the role that superfoods play in our quest to lose weight, presenting themselves as shortcuts to shedding pounds. But no amount of avocados or acai berries can be a substitute for an eating pattern emphasizing fruits and vegetables, whole grains, beans, nuts, seafood, and lean poultry, and minimizing processed and junk foods.

In fairy tales, the false hero is eventually exposed, the true hero prevails, and everyone lives happily ever after. If only we could say the same for the real world of weight loss.

What to Do

➲ Instead of fixating on specific foods, focus on general categories such as vegetables, fruits, beans, seeds, nuts, and fish. Choose foods within those groups based on what you like—not what you think you must eat.

➲ Don't expect that upping your intake of fruits, vegetables, and salads, by itself, will control your weight. What matters is the overall composition of your diet.

➲ Watch out for health halos. Don't assume that foods are weight-friendly just because they carry labels such as "natural," "light," "gluten-free," or "organic," or are sold at farmers' markets.

Chapter 5

TIMING *ISN'T* EVERYTHING

I encounter plenty of diets that make me howl, but none more so than the werewolf diet. Also known as the moon diet or lunar diet, the plan involves timing your eating according to the phases of the moon. For example, during a full moon, solid foods are off-limits. When the moon is waxing, you're supposed to avoid sweets. When it's waning, you need to drink 8 glasses of water a day. Oh, and you must greet the new moon by downing dandelion tea and other "detoxifying" drinks.

Proponents claim that the diet, which orbits around the notion that the moon's gravitational pull affects the water in our bodies, can help you lose up to 6 pounds a day. There's zero evidence for any of this, but that hasn't stopped celebrities like Madonna from reportedly embracing the loony lunar diet.

Though less far-fetched, other weight-loss rules and regimens operate on the same basic principle—that *when* we eat is just as important as *what* we eat. Among the edicts: Always have breakfast. Eat most of your calories early. No fruit after 2 p.m. Have small meals throughout the day. Eat only during an eight-hour window. Never eat anything after

8 p.m. Stop eating at least two hours before bedtime. Don't eat on certain days.

Such approaches to weight loss, which I put under the heading of meal timing, have become more popular in recent years. But the notion that our bodies respond best when fed (or not fed) at certain times isn't new. Traditional Chinese medicine, which goes back thousands of years, asserts that energy from each organ in the body peaks during a two-hour window and that eating should be timed accordingly. For example, the stomach is said to be strongest from 7 to 9 a.m., so that's the time to consume the biggest meal of the day. People should have a light dinner between 5 and 7 p.m., when the kidneys work best. And food should be avoided at night, when digestive organs are at their nadir.

Though organ-specific windows aren't part of Western medicine, the underlying idea—that the body operates according to a 24-hour clock—is widely accepted as a scientific fact. And the effects of this internal clock, or circadian rhythm, on metabolism, appetite, and hormones form the basis for some meal-timing measures to control weight.

The problem is that much of the research on meal timing, while interesting, is far from conclusive. Yet we often hear these directives portrayed as proven ways to lose weight. And we eagerly comply, making sacrifices to do so— whether by forcing ourselves to eat when we're not hungry, forcing ourselves *not* to eat when we *are* hungry, or missing meals with friends and family because they occur at the "wrong" time.

While some people find success with some of these approaches, the truth is that they're not a panacea and should be seen for what they often are: hard-to-follow rules based on soft science.

The Breakfast Serial

For more than 100 years, breakfast has been hailed as the most important meal of the day, and over time, its purported benefits have expanded to include weight control. Much of the credit for breakfast's reputation goes to makers of the quintessential breakfast food—cereal.

The story begins with Dr. John Harvey Kellogg, the most influential health promoter of the early 20th century. Seeking an alternative to meat-heavy breakfasts that were typical at the time, Kellogg and his brother Will created the first ready-to-eat flaked cereal. (Eventually, Will formed his own cereal business, which became the Kellogg Company that exists today.)

A 1917 article in Dr. Kellogg's monthly magazine, *Good Health*, was among the first to extol the virtues of breakfast. "In many ways, the breakfast is the most important meal of the day, because it is the meal that gets the day started," wrote Lenna Frances Cooper, a protégée and employee of Dr. Kellogg's who would become a leader in the field of dietetics. Breakfast, she said, should consist of "easily digested foods" and "not be a heavy meal."

The cereal maker C. W. Post used aggressive marketing to further elevate breakfast's status. Having been a patient at Dr. Kellogg's Battle Creek Sanitarium—a luxurious, world-famous health spa located in Battle Creek, Michigan—Post set up shop nearby to make his own cereal (much to the dismay of the Kelloggs, who accused him of stealing their recipes).

Early ads for Post's first cereal, Grape-Nuts, hawked the product's ability to "begin the day well" by supplying "all the elements for perfect nutrition." A morning bowl of this miracle food could supposedly help children grow, make old people "alert, brisk and vigorous," and keep everyone "strong, well and brainy." One newspaper ad went so far as to call it "the most scientific brain and nerve food in existence."

"Because of his innovative promotional techniques," writes food historian Abigail Carroll in her book *Three Squares*, "Post's influence on the morning meal . . . was profound." Post's advertising shaped not only what people ate, but also what they expected breakfast to do for their health.

By the 1950s, ads for Grape-Nuts were focusing on its alleged impact on weight. One ad, for example, showed a smiling young woman holding a sexy dress against her thin body as a heavier woman glared jealously at her. Another proclaimed that "the trimmest weight watchers just happen to eat Post Grape-Nuts."

The theme continued in a 1960s Grape-Nuts ad campaign featuring a shapely mom named Caroline Burke and her look-alike teenage daughter, Dale. The iconic TV commercial, which spawned numerous parodies, showed a young man mistakenly grabbing Caroline in the swimming pool and then exclaiming, "Oh no, *Mrs.* Burke. I thought you were Dale!" Her secret to staying so slim? Exercise and Grape-Nuts for breakfast. The ad concluded with the slogan "It fills you up, not out."

In the decades that followed, the Kellogg Company reinforced the message about breakfast and weight through ads for Special K, which, like those for Grape-Nuts, targeted mainly women. Among the most memorable catchphrases was "you can't pinch an inch." Said one commercial: "If you can pinch an inch"—and who can't?—"the Kellogg's Special K breakfast may help you lose weight."

Likewise, the Special K Challenge ad campaign promised that consuming the cereal for breakfast and one other meal every day could lead to the loss of up to 6 pounds or a jeans size in two weeks. Kellogg's could point to published research supporting the claim—which the company happened to fund.

Indeed, financial support for breakfast-related studies by companies such as Kellogg's and General Mills (whose products include Cheerios, Wheaties, and Total) is commonplace and another way that cereal makers have shaped our perceptions of the morning meal.

Take, for example, an influential study published in the *Journal of the American College of Nutrition*. Analyzing responses from more than 16,000 adults in the US National Health and Nutrition Examination Survey, the researchers concluded that skipping breakfast is associated with higher weight and eating cereal is linked to lower weight. The study, which has been cited more than 500 times, was not only funded by Kellogg's; the company also helped conduct it.

Other observational studies, some industry-funded and some not, have likewise found that breakfast eaters tend to weigh less than breakfast skippers. The most common explanation is that forgoing breakfast increases hunger, causing people to overeat later.

Sounds plausible, but these studies show only associations, not cause and effect. It could be that breakfast eaters are thinner because of other lifestyle habits or traits that research didn't account for.

Sorting this out requires randomized trials, the type of studies that can show cause and effect. And in such research, breakfast has come up short. Pooling results from seven trials, researchers found that those assigned to eat breakfast did not lose more weight. Nor did they consume fewer calories. In fact, breakfast eaters on average took in 260 *more* calories per day than breakfast skippers. The study concluded that "caution is needed when recommending breakfast for weight loss in adults, as it could have the opposite effect."

Of course, not all breakfasts are equal. Starting your day with glazed doughnuts or a bowl of Cocoa Krispies is not the same as eating steel-cut oats and blueberries. By focusing more on *whether* people ate than *what* they ate, breakfast studies have generally failed to take such differences into account. So it could be that certain types of breakfasts—those made up of healthful, filling foods, for example—do help with weight loss, while others don't. But at this point, there's insufficient evidence to know for certain.

What we can say is that the oft-repeated axiom that you must eat breakfast to lose weight is unproven. In fact, there's evidence refuting it. When led to believe the standard line, those who prefer to skip breakfast may needlessly force down food they don't want and wind up eating more than they otherwise would have. Not exactly a recipe for effective weight loss—or pleasant mornings.

On the other hand, if you enjoy breakfast, as I do, it's perfectly fine to eat, as long as you're mindful of what you put on your plate or in your bowl. For me, that's whole grain cereal, a choice that would surely please both Dr. Kellogg and Mr. Post.

MYTH OR TRUTH?

Exercising before breakfast leads to greater weight loss.

The idea behind exercising on an empty stomach—a practice sometimes called "fasted cardio"—is that when stored carbohydrate in the body is depleted because we haven't eaten, we burn mainly fat. Indeed, there's some evidence that fasted cardio may boost fat burning, but only fleetingly. Over the course of days or weeks, which is what counts, fasted cardio doesn't appear to promote loss of either fat or weight in general. For example, a six-week study involving overweight women who did high-intensity interval workouts after either fasting or eating found no differences in body composition. In a review of this and other studies, researchers concluded that pre-breakfast exercise is no more effective for losing fat or weight. For many of us, exercising on an empty stomach is like driving a car with no gas. Eating a light breakfast beforehand can supply the energy we need to keep moving.

Night Moves

Whether or not we eat breakfast, we increasingly hear that we should consume most of our calories earlier in the day in order to lose weight. Sometimes this guidance takes the form of a rule to move up dinnertime or not eat after a particular hour at night. Consistent with the old adage "Eat breakfast like a king, lunch like a prince, and dinner like a pauper," the prevailing wisdom exhorts us to avoid big meals in the evening.

Pushed by some weight-loss gurus and diet plans, the "eat earlier" mantra is trumpeted in articles with headlines such as "When Trying to Lose Weight, Morning Meals Are Better Than Evening Ones" and "Why Eating Late at Night May Be Particularly Bad for You and Your Diet."

Typically the explanations involve our circadian rhythms and their influence on how our bodies respond to food. For example, we burn fewer calories digesting food in the evening than in the morning. In addition, our cells are less sensitive to the hormone insulin at night, which means higher blood sugar levels and possibly more fat accumulation. But it's unclear how much these and other circadian variations actually matter when it comes to our weight.

Some, but not all, observational studies show a correlation between later eating and higher weight. For example, in a study of Italians who were followed for six years, those who consumed at least half their daily calories at dinner were more than twice as likely to become obese as those who got less than a third of their calories from the evening meal. Both groups took in about the same number of calories throughout the day.

Such research doesn't prove cause and effect, however. As for randomized trials, one of the most frequently cited is an Israeli study involving 74 overweight women. They were assigned one of two meal plans with identical calorie counts: a breakfast-dominant diet consisting of 700 calories for breakfast, 500 for lunch, and 200 for dinner; or a dinner-dominant diet that flipped calorie counts for breakfast and dinner and kept lunch the same. After 12 weeks, people in both groups lost weight—but those eating the lighter dinner shed about 11 pounds more on average.

Since the study was short term, though, we don't know whether front-loading calories is beneficial over the long run. What's more, other randomized studies have failed to show any effect at all. When researchers pooled results from the Israeli trial and four others, they found no difference between smaller and larger dinners when it came to weight. "Recommendations to reduce evening intake," they wrote, "cannot be substantiated by clinical evidence."

In addition to the lack of solid proof, lots of unanswered questions surround the recommendations. For example, what percentage of calories at night is optimal? How early should most calories be consumed? And how late is too late to eat? For someone living in the US, an 8 p.m. dinnertime may be "late." But someone in Spain would consider that early.

Likewise, are some people more susceptible to the effects of later eating because of their genetics or circadian rhythms? Some research suggests, for instance, that those with a so-called late chronotype—a.k.a. night owls—may be more likely to gain weight from nighttime eating than early-to-bed types. But such findings are preliminary.

In short, there are too many unknowns to draw any firm conclusions. And there's a potential downside to the ban on nighttime eating: Time-strapped people facing an early-dinner deadline may be more likely to rely on vending machines or fast-food drive-throughs for their evening meals. If early eating leads in such ways to unhealthy food choices, it's better to wait until later, when there's time for a more healthful meal.

Regardless of whether circadian variations play a role, it's true that after-dinner snacking can pose a problem. Mindlessly munching on chips in front of the TV or raiding the refrigerator for leftover pizza leads to extra calories and possibly extra pounds. The same goes for polishing off that pint of ice cream because of tiredness or stress, both of which may contribute to nighttime munchies.

To avoid such temptations, some people find it helpful to "close the kitchen" and stop eating after dinner. Or if you're truly hungry, go for a light, satisfying snack such as plain yogurt, a hard-boiled egg, or carrots and hummus.

For most of us, these steps are easier to follow than trying to align eating with our circadian rhythms. And, given the iffy evidence, they're also a surer bet for weight control.

MYTH OR TRUTH?

You shouldn't eat protein and carbohydrates at the same time.

Food combining, the practice of eating certain foods separately, has been around for thousands of years as part of the ancient healing system from India known as Ayurveda. In the

1920s, Dr. William Howard Hay popularized food combining as a remedy for weight control, and since then it's been a feature of many diet plans. Though the rules can get complicated, the basic concept is to avoid eating carbs and protein in the same meal. Also, fruit should be eaten only on an empty stomach. Supposedly, mixing the "wrong" foods inhibits proper digestion and allows undigested food to rot in the stomach, leading to weight gain. All this is unscientific hokum, however, and ignores the fact that many foods from beans to bread contain a combination of protein and carbs. The little research that exists has found that a food-combining diet produces no greater weight loss than a regular diet with the same number of calories. If someone does shed pounds on a food-combining regimen, it's because of what and how much they ate, not when they ate it.

Life in the Fast Lane

Fasting is, in many ways, the granddaddy of meal-timing strategies. It has certainly been around a long time: The ancient Greek physician Hippocrates extolled its virtues, as did Plato and Aristotle. Many religious traditions embrace the practice, with the faithful from Mormons to Muslims abstaining from eating and drinking at certain times.

It has also been the subject of considerable research—mainly in animals—which suggests that fasting may help protect against conditions such as heart disease, cancer, and diabetes; improve brain function; and increase longevity. But most of the buzz relates to its purported power as a weight-loss tactic, a reputation undoubtedly enhanced by testimonials from celebrities such as Jennifer Aniston and Jimmy Kimmel.

The form they promote—intermittent fasting (IF)—is an umbrella term for several different approaches: time-restricted feeding, which entails eating only during a limited window and then fasting the rest of the day; alternate-day fasting, in which you consume 500 or fewer calories every other day; and the 5:2 diet, in which you similarly restrict calories on two nonconsecutive days each week.

Proponents point out that our hunter-gatherer ancestors didn't eat three meals a day. They regularly had to survive without eating when food was scarce, so thanks to evolution, our bodies are well equipped to handle little or no food for long periods.

One feature making this possible is our ability to tap stored fat for energy when we're deprived of glucose from food. It's thought that this extra fat burning may lead to weight loss when people fast—the same principle behind forgoing carbs on the keto diet. Of course it's also possible that people drop pounds when fasting simply because they take in fewer calories.

Whatever the reason, studies do show that IF is effective for weight loss—but not more so than standard calorie-cutting diets. In one study, for example, researchers assigned 100 obese participants to either an alternate-day fasting diet, a calorie-reduced diet, or a control group with no dietary restrictions. After six months, people on the fasting and calorie-reduction regimens fared exactly the same, losing about 7 percent more of their body weight, on average, than the controls. During the next six months, both diet groups regained some weight, and again the amounts were virtually identical.

A larger trial of more than 300 participants found that those assigned to IF actually lost a bit *less* weight after a year than subjects on a calorie-restricted diet—11 pounds versus 15—though the difference wasn't statistically significant. A number of smaller head-to-head comparisons have also shown no difference in outcomes.

Going without food for long stretches is, to say the least, a challenge for many of us. And, as with other diets, a key question is how sustainable IF regimens are. In some studies, dropout rates have been relatively high. Other studies have found dropout rates to be comparable to those of calorie-reduced diets, though that's not exactly a ringing endorsement. And since most IF studies have lasted less than a year, we don't know about long-term adherence.

Another unknown is whether some types of IF regimens are more effective than others. Most studies to date have involved fasting for 24 hours (whether on alternate days or two days a week) rather than time-restricted feeding. It could be that squeezing all our eating into a narrow window yields better results than other IF approaches, but given the limited evidence, that's just speculation.

Likewise, science doesn't provide clear answers about how long the window should be or at what hours it should occur for optimal results. But that hasn't stopped all kinds of "experts" from issuing definitive-sounding rules about when to begin and end your fast each day.

Enthusiasts also tend to gloss over the potential risks. Being deprived of food for long periods may lead to overeating during non-fasting times, which could be a problem especially for those prone to binge eating. Similarly, the severe restrictions make IF a bad idea for anyone with a history of eating disorders such as anorexia. The same goes for pregnant women or people who take certain medications.

What's more, there's some evidence that IF induces a greater loss of lean mass (which includes muscle) than conventional calorie-restricted diets. That's important because the goal of any regimen should be to maximize fat loss while preserving muscle, which burns more calories than fat and helps protect us from disability as we age.

Another major drawback of IF is the potential sacrifice required. Meals are often about more than eating, after all. They're an important way that we socialize with friends and loved ones, an opportunity to enjoy food and the company of others. Fasting regimens may force us to miss out on this great pleasure in life.

All these downsides seem a high price to pay for weight loss that is probably no greater than what you achieve with other diets and isn't proven to last long term. While IF, like other regimens, may work well for certain people, for many others it's just another road to frustration and failure. Despite the promises of those beckoning us to take this route, we should heed the flashing yellow lights.

Kevin's Journey

Kevin had been a personal trainer for years. So when it came to managing his weight, he knew the right combination of nutrition and exercise to maintain the physique he wanted. But a few years ago, the techniques he had relied on started to fail him.

At the time, Kevin was working as a chef, which was a recipe for weight gain. He was in a job that involved being around food all day and didn't provide the same opportunities for physical activity as personal training had.

Having difficulty battling the extra pounds, Kevin resorted to techniques he never would have considered before. Among them: intermittent fasting. He recalls doing some Internet research on IF, which generated a constant stream of content about the subject on his Facebook feed. Maybe the subliminal messaging got to him, or perhaps he really thought fasting would work. Whatever the reason, Kevin soon downloaded an app to his phone that would start to control his life.

The app called for a rotating schedule of fasting periods on different days—from a low of 12 hours of fasting to a high of 20—with two days off each week. Kevin set his schedule so that he'd eat in the evening after work. "I sleep for eight of those hours, so how hard can it be?" he thought. In fact, hunger was not an issue, but the routine did create other problems that would prove insurmountable.

Kevin found himself watching the clock all day in anticipation of his allowed mealtime. "It got into my head," he says. And when it came time to eat, the only foods he wanted were ones filled with salt and sugar, like chips and candied fruits, instead of the balanced meals that he knew were good for him.

In addition, he worked out less because he lacked energy, and he found it difficult to balance his social life with a fasting routine, since gatherings with friends and family often involve food. Contrary to what Kevin had read about IF, it didn't sharpen his mind. If anything, it created the sense that he was punishing himself. And, worst of all, he didn't lose weight.

Kevin tried IF on and off a few times before concluding that it didn't work for him and wasn't sustainable. Today, he has returned to his tried-and-true recipes: focusing on protein and vegetables, and cutting back on alcohol. And with the encouragement of his new workout buddy—his pit bull and Lab mix, Delilah—he's getting the exercise he needs. Though Kevin no longer follows a strict eating schedule, he's happy to accommodate Delilah's walking schedule.

Mini-Meals

In contrast to fasting, which narrows eating opportunities, there's another meal-timing strategy that does just the opposite. I'm referring to grazing, which involves having multiple small meals a day—typically every two to three hours—instead of the standard three.

While most of us were taught that we're supposed to eat three times a day, that number isn't based on biological needs. Instead, it's a function of culture and tradition. Throughout history, the norm has varied, with some societies consuming fewer than three meals a day and others eating more.

For still others, the concept of meals as we define them didn't even exist. For example, when European settlers arrived in America, they discovered that Native people didn't eat according to a set schedule but instead were guided by hunger and the availability of food. The Europeans considered this practice uncivilized, though as historian Abigail

Carroll observed, the colonists' haphazard eating habits might be judged similarly by today's standards.

Given that meal frequency is a cultural construct, there's nothing inherently wrong or unnatural about eating, say, six times a day instead of three. The question for our purposes is whether it's more effective at controlling weight, as proponents claim.

Their explanation is that frequent eating reduces hunger, helping us eat less overall. Also, it supposedly boosts metabolism because digesting the extra meals takes extra energy.

Some observational studies do show that people who eat more frequent meals are less likely to be overweight. But other research has linked greater frequency with *higher* weight or found no association.

The results of experimental studies are even less compelling. In one study, for instance, researchers assigned 51 subjects either to eat three meals a day or to graze by consuming at least 100 calories every two to three hours. All participants were instructed to get the same total number of daily calories. After six months, both groups lost weight, but on average, the amounts were the same. Virtually all other trials have also failed to show any advantage of grazing.

In addition, the case that grazing speeds metabolism is unproven. But there is some support for the claim that it helps control hunger. In the aforementioned study finding no greater weight loss among grazers, they nevertheless did experience a decline in hunger, while those who ate three meals did not.

So if frequent eaters are less hungry, why don't they shed more pounds? For some people, the more often they're exposed to food, the more they eat, regardless of hunger level. Plus, as discussed in chapter 2, we tend to underestimate the number of calories in foods, so eating more frequently means more opportunities to overdo it. The result of this one-two punch is that grazing may not deliver on weight loss as promised, and for some, it can add up to weight gain.

As with other meal-timing approaches, *what* you eat is key. Grazing on whole foods like fruits, vegetables, and legumes is more likely to help peel off pounds than relying on processed foods like chips and candy bars. If you're at work all day with limited access to healthy foods, grazing may not be a good option. Ditto if you're at home with a pantry full of tempting junk food.

Personality and preferences also play a role. If you tend to be a grazer and are able to control the amount you consume, frequent eating may indeed be a winning strategy. But if you prefer three (or fewer) meals a day or have trouble keeping portions limited, then grazing isn't likely to help you.

In short, whether frequent eating is right for you depends on a number of factors. And even if it is right, it may not be any more effective at controlling your weight. As with all sales offers, the pitch for grazing comes with terms and conditions. Unfortunately, the sellers too often fail to show us the fine print.

MYTH OR TRUTH?

Snacking between meals affects your weight.

Though there's overlap between snacking and grazing, the practices, as I define them, are different. With grazing, people eat multiple mini-meals *instead* of the standard three a day, while snacks are consumed *in addition* to those three squares. Some experts warn that eating between meals undermines weight control, but others say it can help. In fact, the research doesn't provide clear answers either way.

Snacking's effects likely depend on what we eat and how filling it is. Snacks that are higher in fiber and protein—apple slices with peanut butter, for example—may help prevent hunger and overeating. But foods like cookies and pretzels are likely to leave you hungry. Portion sizes and calories also matter, as does why you're snacking. If you're doing so mindfully and strategically to control hunger, snacking may be beneficial. But if you're snacking because you're bored or stressed, or because you can't resist those doughnuts in the break room at work, the extra food can wind up adding extra pounds.

No Easy Time

Whether it's eating breakfast, avoiding late meals, fasting, or grazing, *when* we eat may indeed play a role in weight control for some people. But we don't know which people are most likely to benefit, which measures are most likely to help, or how much they can help.

As a result, if you want to try meal timing, you're flying blind to a large extent. Now, that's not necessarily a bad thing. Many endeavors in life, including weight loss, require trial and error. But before taking off, we need to be aware of the unknowns and possible downsides, and too often we aren't.

Frequently people go in with unrealistic expectations because of friends or celebrities who rave about their amazing results, or weight-loss gurus who overstate the evidence and downplay the drawbacks. Even scientists sometimes lead us astray. For example, when one researcher was interviewed about her study showing that time-restricted feeding leads to short-term weight loss, she gushed, "It's so simple. All you have to do is watch the clock."

The truth is that adhering to a strict timetable governing when you eat or don't eat is often far from simple. It can require enormous self-discipline and effort, a task made even harder by the demands of daily life. That's why meal-timing regimens may be tough to sustain for more than a few weeks or months. And even if we can stick with them, these strategies may yield little or no benefit.

If we're not fully prepared for these possibilities, we may feel guilt or shame when we deviate from the schedule. And if we don't see the promised results, we may blame ourselves, wrongly concluding that our lack of willpower is the problem when in fact the regimens are.

As previously discussed, these negative feelings are the same ones that people experience when restrictive diets and calorie counting fail. Though we often hear that meal-timing regimens are superior to these other approaches, it turns out they're often just another version of the same thing: a one-size-fits-all "solution" that works for some people in the short term but is hard to sustain and isn't a long-term answer.

The alternative is the same as well: finding what's right for you based on your own preferences and needs. That may include breakfast or not. It may mean dinner at 5 p.m. or 9 p.m. or somewhere in between. And it may involve eating once a day or three times or six.

The key is to choose foods you like that are healthful and filling, and enjoy them on a schedule aligned with what your body tells you, what makes you feel good, and what's doable given the requirements of work, family, and everyday life.

A meal-timing schedule that's imposed on us in the absence of these considerations is like a clock that's always wrong. If we rely on it, we're certain to have trouble staying on track.

What to Do

⮑ If intermittent fasting or other meal-timing strategies are effective for you, it's okay to keep doing them. But if they make life difficult or don't work, don't blame yourself.

⮑ Time your eating according to your preferences and schedule. There are no across-the-board answers to whether to eat breakfast, when to eat dinner, how many meals a day are optimal, or how long to refrain from eating.

⮑ Try to keep after-dinner eating to a minimum. If you're truly hungry, go for a light, healthy snack.

Chapter 6

BOTTLED BUNK

It was a medical miracle. Or so it seemed. In 1933, Stanford University physicians published research in the *Journal of the American Medical Association* showing that a drug could boost metabolism by 50 percent, melting away 20 pounds in 10 weeks—with no dieting.

As word of the remarkable findings spread, demand for the drug skyrocketed. Soon, more than 20 companies were selling it in over-the-counter products with names like Slim, Corpu-Lean, and Formula 281. (Too-weighty one. Get it?) By 1934, at least 100,000 people in the US had taken the drug.

As its popularity grew, so did reports of side effects. Among them: rashes, numbness, yellowing of the skin and eyes, and blindness due to cataracts. And there was this one too: death. The drug overheated users, sometimes so much that it caused cardiac arrest. Basically, they were broiled on the inside, which is not a pleasant way to go.

The fact that the drug, a chemical called 2,4-dinitrophenol, or DNP, could be dangerous was no surprise. Here's the first clue: It's an explosive that was used to make weapons. When French munitions workers absorbed DNP through their skin and lungs during World War I, some fell ill and died. The workers also tended to lose weight, which led to the Stanford doctors' not-so-bright idea that swallowing the stuff—albeit only under a physician's supervision, which they incorrectly believed would make it safe—could be a good way to combat obesity.

The American Medical Association disagreed, declaring that treating obesity "with a toxic agent capable of inducing serious injury and death appears to be unjustified." As reports of side effects mounted in the 1930s, US federal regulators grew increasingly alarmed, but the laws at the time severely limited their powers to act.

That changed in 1938, when Congress passed legislation expanding the authority of both the FDA and the Federal Trade Commission (FTC). The newly empowered officials wasted no time in ordering DNP to be removed from drugstore shelves and labeling it "unfit for human consumption."

This should have ended the sad saga of DNP's use as a weight-loss remedy. But alas, the drug is now back. Though DNP is banned for use in medications and dietary supplements, various manufacturers peddle it on the Internet as a "fat burner" supplement for bodybuilders and dieters.

Tragically, DNP is once again claiming lives. A number of DNP-related deaths have been reported in recent years, mainly among young people in the US and the United Kingdom. And once again, regulators are unable to stop the sale of DNP. Though the FDA has gone after some sellers, it's playing a game of whack-a-mole. DNP hucksters, who often operate outside the US, have managed to stay a step ahead of the outgunned authorities.

DNP isn't the only illegal and potentially harmful ingredient showing up in dietary supplements for weight loss. A number of products have been found to contain the prescription appetite suppressant sibutramine (brand name Meridia), which was taken off the US market in 2010 after being found to increase the risk of heart attacks and strokes. Others include the stimulants ephedra and DMAA, both of which have been linked to serious side effects and deaths, and banned for use in dietary supplements.

As for the legal ingredients in weight-loss supplements, most have unknown risks and unproven benefits because the government doesn't require manufacturers to test their products or provide evidence of safety and effectiveness. Nor is there any guarantee that supplements contain the amounts of ingredients listed on the label. And as I mentioned, they may contain ingredients that aren't listed.

Nevertheless, Americans wager more than $6 billion annually on weight-loss supplements in hopes of finding a magic bullet that will make unwanted pounds disappear without serious side effects. It's a bet—prompted by our desire for quick fixes, egged on by deceptive marketing, and made possible by lax regulation—that we keep losing.

Iffy Ingredients

Weight-loss supplements typically contain a hodgepodge of ingredients. The most common is caffeine, which sometimes comes in the form of herbs such as guarana, kola nut, or yerba maté. As a stimulant, caffeine can modestly boost metabolism and fat burning, but it's unclear whether the effects are large enough to result in weight loss.

In a frequently cited study on caffeine and weight, researchers followed more than 58,000 health professionals for 12 years, estimating their caffeine intake based on diet questionnaires. Overall, participants put on weight during the period, but those who upped their caffeine consumption gained a pound or so less than those whose caffeine intake went down. Hardly anything to write home about. Plus, because the study was observational, it's possible the findings were due to something other than caffeine.

Surprisingly, there are few randomized trials examining how caffeine affects weight loss. The ones that exist are small and usually combine caffeine with other substances, making it difficult to tease out the effects of caffeine. Randomized studies testing the claim that it can curb appetite and make us eat less have yielded mixed results.

The extent to which caffeine influences metabolism and weight may depend on several factors, including how much we routinely consume. Heavy users are less likely to be affected by caffeine because their bodies have built up a tolerance to it. The dose also matters, as does what caffeine is combined with. Pairing it with other stimulants, as weight-loss supplements sometimes do, can have synergistic effects.

Such combinations—for example, caffeine plus ephedra—can be dangerous. So can high doses of caffeine. (The safe upper limit for most adults is 400 milligrams, the amount in 3 or 4 cups of coffee.) In a study of adverse events reported to the FDA, weight-loss supplements containing caffeine were more likely than products without caffeine to be associated with severe side effects such as hospitalizations and deaths.

Green tea extract, another common ingredient in weight-loss supplements, typically contains caffeine along with antioxidants known as catechins. The most abundant catechin in green tea, epigallocatechin gallate, or EGCG, often gets star billing. Proponents claim that the combination of EGCG and caffeine, which research suggests may ramp up metabolism and fat burning more than caffeine alone, is key to green tea extract's alleged power to peel away pounds.

But studies overall have failed to show much, if any, effect on weight. When researchers pooled results from seven trials, they found green tea extract to be no better than a placebo.

Another review of studies concluded that any weight loss is "very small" and "not likely . . . clinically important."

As for safety, products containing green tea extract have been linked to liver damage. The risk is thought to be greatest when people ingest the substance on an empty stomach. (Drinking moderate amounts of green tea doesn't pose this danger.)

The discussion of tea leads us to coffee—or specifically green coffee bean extract, a common ingredient in weight-loss supplements that was popularized by Dr. Oz. (More on that later.) *Green* coffee beans are ones that haven't been roasted. They're higher than roasted beans in a compound called chlorogenic acid, which some research suggests may have a beneficial effect on weight. Like green tea and roasted beans, green coffee beans contain caffeine as well.

In a review of 15 randomized trials, Iranian researchers found that green coffee extract produced greater weight loss than a placebo. But the difference—less than 3 pounds—was minimal. All the studies were small and short term, and most were of poor quality. Another review concluded that because of methodological shortcomings in the research, "green coffee extract is not recommended as a safe or effective treatment for weight loss."

The list of other ingredients in weight-loss supplements is endless, with new ones appearing all the time. Some claim to work by boosting metabolism, while others supposedly suppress appetite, affect the formation or breakdown of fat, or block the absorption of carbohydrates or fat from foods. It's practically impossible to cover all the ingredients that show up in products, but here's the lowdown on seven that manufacturers frequently include.

- **Carnitine:** A substance produced by the body and found in foods, especially red meat. Some trials show a very small effect on weight loss, which decreases over time. There are hints—but no hard proof—that carnitine may be associated with an elevated risk of cardiovascular disease.

➲ **Chromium:** A mineral, typically in the form of chromium picolinate in supplements. Some studies have found that it leads to lower weight, but just barely. One review calls the evidence "insufficient" to support its use for weight loss.

➲ **CLA:** A fatty acid found mainly in beef and dairy products. In a few studies, there was a small effect on weight, but other trials—including those of higher quality—turned up no improvement.

➲ **Forskolin:** A compound from the roots of *Coleus forskohlii*, a plant from the mint family. There are only a few trials, all of which are small, and results are inconsistent.

➲ ***Garcinia cambogia:*** A substance from a fruit-bearing tree native to Asia and Africa. The rind contains the compound hydroxycitric acid, which is thought to be the active ingredient. A few studies have found effects on weight, while others show none. Products containing *Garcinia cambogia* have been linked to liver damage and psychiatric disorders, though it's possible other ingredients may have played a role.

➲ **Glucomannan:** A soluble fiber derived from the root of the konjac plant. It absorbs up to 50 times its weight in water, which may help users feel full. Overall, research is mixed about its effect on weight. An analysis pooling results from eight trials found no effect.

⊃ **Raspberry ketone:** A compound found in raspberries that's used as a flavoring agent. There's
virtually no evidence from human trials to support its use for weight loss. Some researchers
warn that high doses may have harmful effects
on the heart.

Overall, what we can say from the limited evidence is that
a few ingredients in supplements *may* lead to a few pounds of
weight loss in the short run, but we don't know whether they
help long term. Adding further to the uncertainty, levels of
ingredients vary from product to product and aren't always
disclosed, with some labels unhelpfully referring only to a
"proprietary blend." What's more, it's often unclear how combining a particular ingredient with multiple substances, as
supplements typically do, influences effectiveness.

The same goes for safety. While the available evidence
may suggest that an ingredient has few or no side effects
when used alone, what happens when it's combined with
other ingredients? It's quite possible that some compounds
interact in ways that are harmful. But because there hasn't
been rigorous—or in some cases any—testing, there's no
way to tell.

What we do know is that certain ingredients can interact
with prescription medications. For example, carnitine may
reduce the effectiveness of thyroid replacement hormones.
Chromium picolinate, when combined with diabetes medicines, may lead to low blood sugar. And forskolin may interfere with the blood-thinning drug warfarin. But supplement
labels typically don't disclose such information.

In short, taking a supplement for weight loss is a leap in
the dark. If the products had to meet the same standards of
proof for safety and effectiveness as medications, few, if any,
would be allowed on the market.

MYTH OR TRUTH?

Protein powder helps you lose weight.

Protein is often promoted for weight loss because it helps fill us up and may decrease hunger. In addition, our bodies expend more energy digesting protein than carbs or fat. Overall, studies suggest that in the short term, eating more protein (while keeping total calories the same) may modestly enhance weight loss while preserving more muscle mass. But findings are mixed on whether extra protein helps over the long run. In one study, for example, 150 people who had lost weight were randomly assigned to consume at each meal one of three protein powders—whey, whey plus calcium, or soy—or a powder devoid of protein. (The powders were mixed into shakes or soups.) After six months, all groups had regained the same amount of weight.

Though powders can be a convenient way to get extra protein, there's nothing magical about them. Sprinkling them into a 600-calorie sugary smoothie, for instance, won't turn it into a weight-friendly food. But protein powder may be beneficial if it's used for shakes that replace snacks or added to foods such as oatmeal to help fill you up.

Same Old Song and Dance

In 1914, an article in *Good Housekeeping* decried the plethora of weight-loss remedies that were worthless or dangerous, and the deceptive techniques used to sell them. Titled "Swindled Getting Slim," the exposé—coauthored by Dr. Harvey Wiley, a tireless crusader for safe foods and drugs whose efforts led to the creation of the FDA—revealed the ingenuity of marketers "in presenting simple old-time frauds under new names . . . with marvelous scientific explanations as to how they do the work, and new assurances of harmlessness and effectiveness."

The sellers of these mail-order products, said the article, "are getting richer every day that a complaisant government allows their advertisements."

Such ads claimed that weight-loss pills were "prepared scientifically" to "quickly remove" fat with "no dieting—no exercise." The remedies were "perfectly safe" and came with "guaranteed" satisfaction or your money back.

Fast-forwarding to today, weight-loss supplements are promoted as "scientifically formulated" to provide "immediate results" and "burn more calories without diet or exercise." They advertise "no side effects" and a 30-day money-back guarantee.

Dr. Wiley would be disheartened to see how little things have changed.

Dietary supplements are regulated under a 1994 law known as the Dietary Supplement Health and Education Act (DSHEA). While it forbids manufacturers to claim that a product can treat, prevent, or cure a disease, DSHEA does allow them to say a supplement "maintains," "supports," or "promotes" normal functioning—a distinction that's largely meaningless to the average consumer.

Basically, the law assumes that supplements are innocent until proven guilty—just the opposite of how medications are regulated. Rather than requiring manufacturers to demonstrate that their products are safe and effective prior to marketing, DSHEA puts the burden on the FDA to prove that a supplement is dangerous and should be taken off the market—a process that often requires lengthy legal battles.

Supplement advertising falls under the jurisdiction of the FTC. Stopping deceptive ads also entails legal action, and the FTC lacks the resources to go after the vast majority of offenders.

A few have been caught, however, and in some cases forced to pay fines. Among the campaigns the FTC has targeted:

- ➲ "Get high school skinny." This was the tagline for ads claiming that a brand of supplements could shave off as much as 165 pounds without changes in diet or lifestyle. One of the company's cofounders, who was featured in radio ads and TV infomercials, agreed to be banned from the weight-loss industry. But the products are still on the market (with more restrained claims), and promotional videos featuring the cofounder are still on YouTube.

- ➲ "You can keep eating your favorite foods and STILL lose pounds and inches; in fact we guarantee it!" This was one of several over-the-top claims for two brands of supplements sold by a husband-and-wife team who were also accused of failing to fully disclose the terms of their "risk-free" trial. After customers signed up, the vendor charged their credit cards $80 and continued to collect monthly payments without their consent. Returns and cancellations were difficult.

- ➲ "Hi! CNN says this is one of the best." This was a spam e-mail that sellers used to hawk forskolin and other weight-loss supplements. First, they paid for e-mails to be sent to consumers from hacked accounts, making it seem that the messages came from the users' contacts. The e-mails lured consumers to click links to websites that appeared to be from news sources but weren't. These phony news sites included testimonials from people claiming to have lost 4 pounds a week, as well as fake endorsements by Oprah Winfrey.

➲ "Lost an average of 10% of their body weight without changing diet or exercise." This was the dubious claim in a press release put out by a company selling green coffee bean extract. Initially, the company hired a researcher in India to conduct a trial on its extract. The trial was poorly done and unpublishable, so the company paid two University of Scranton professors to rewrite the study. They concluded that participants who consumed green coffee bean lost an average of 18 pounds. The research was published, and Dr. Oz hailed the study on his program, asking, "Could this be the magic weight-loss bean to help melt away unwanted pounds?" Capitalizing on Oz's adulation for green coffee extract, the company issued the press release highlighting the "staggering" findings. But the FTC said the company "knew or should have known that this botched study didn't prove anything." Eventually, the study was retracted.

While such cases represent a tiny portion of offenses—most escape detection and punishment by the FTC—they nevertheless illustrate some common tactics used to mislead us about weight-loss supplements. The most basic is overblown language about how much weight you will lose, how quickly you'll lose it, or how it's possible to lose it without changing your eating habits. Frequently the promotions also feature images of beautiful models with perfect bodies, which misleadingly imply that you, too, will have a flat stomach and thin thighs if you take the supplement.

Before-and-after photos of satisfied customers are common as well. But these often don't represent most users' experiences. Or they may be photoshopped or completely fabricated. Testimonials, including reviews that appear on Amazon, may also be fake. The same goes for celebrity endorsements.

In addition, makers frequently hype weight-loss supplements as "clinically proven." Typically this refers to research, often unpublished, that is funded by manufacturers for marketing purposes and doesn't provide real proof of effectiveness. In some cases, such studies are conducted only in test tubes or lab animals. In other cases, they're small, short-term human experiments using shoddy methodology. In still others, the research doesn't test that particular supplement but instead involves just components of it, perhaps at a different dose, or other products containing other ingredients.

Marketers also try to bolster scientific credibility by featuring endorsements from doctors or scientists. But these experts, who are paid by manufacturers, are hardly objective, and some have highly questionable credentials.

Using technical terms like *thermogenic, lipolysis*, or *ketosis* to explain how weight-loss supplements supposedly work is another technique that provides a veneer of scientific credibility. The same is true for the use of fancy-sounding, pharmaceutical-like names of proprietary ingredients, which often consist of nothing more than caffeine, coffee bean, or other commonly used substances.

When it comes to safety, supplement sellers try to reassure us by emphasizing that their products are "natural." But keep in mind that while ads may show images of plants or fruits in their natural state, what supplements actually contain often comes from a factory, not the fields. For example, raspberry ketone in supplements is not extracted from raspberries because that process would require huge numbers of berries and would cost too much. Instead, the compound is manufactured in a lab. The amounts that wind up in supplements can be at least 100 times greater than what you'd get in a pound of raspberries and haven't been subjected to rigorous safety testing.

Even if supplement ingredients come directly from nature in relatively small amounts, that's no guarantee that they're safe. Hemlock, after all, is natural, and so are poisonous mushrooms.

The notion that weight-loss supplements can be both highly effective and risk-free—one that often underlies sales pitches—defies basic laws of biology. If a substance is strong enough to meaningfully alter metabolism, fat burning, or other functions, it's also strong enough to cause side effects, at least in some people. The fact that it's "natural" doesn't change this reality.

To be clear, my point is not that all supplements are worthless or harmful, or that all supplement makers are dishonest. Research does show that supplements, from vitamins to fish oil, can be beneficial for certain conditions, and there are plenty of reputable companies that sell them. But when it comes to weight loss, the unfortunate truth is that products generally offer little or no benefit, and the market is awash with shady sellers. We're being bamboozled, and a weak regulatory system is failing to adequately protect us.

Jeremiah's Journey

When Jeremiah walked into a nutrition store, he was seeking a quick fix for a lifelong problem.

One of seven siblings, Jeremiah grew up in a household that prized quantity over quality when it came to food. Frozen dinners, fast food, and mayonnaise sandwiches—Jeremiah's favorite—were the norm. The family celebrated every occasion or achievement with meals that were heavy on fat, carbs, and sugar. Jeremiah calls it "living to eat." He and his entire immediate family were overweight.

When he was a kid, Jeremiah's size made it hard to keep up physically with his peers, who frequently picked on him. The taunting contributed to his sense of shame about his body. He wore baggy clothes to disguise his physique and never took off his shirt around anyone who wasn't part of his family.

In his midteens, Jeremiah decided he had to do something to shed pounds. Diet pills seemed like an ideal solution: take some capsules and watch the excess weight disappear. At least that's what the ads suggested.

When he walked into that nutrition store, he was there to buy a bottle of raspberry ketone, a substance he had seen advertised. Promotions for the supplement said nothing about eating habits, and Jeremiah expected it to melt away pounds as he continued to consume a diet of candy bars, energy drinks, and other junk food. But the supplement failed to deliver as promised, and Jeremiah experienced no noticeable weight loss.

After a short time, he ditched the pills and tried other quick-fix measures, including sleeping in a garbage bag. (Yes, it's a thing. It's dangerous, and it doesn't work.) When those proved ineffective, Jeremiah returned to the supplement store. This time he opted for a multi-pill "fat burner" supplement that ended up providing a burst of energy followed by a crash—but no weight loss. He blamed himself for the failure. "I remember looking at myself in the mirror in disgust," he says, "which led to self-hatred. I beat myself up a lot."

After moving with his wife to another state for her job, the couple separated. This life crisis prompted Jeremiah to tackle his weight problem in a healthier way.

He had come across credible nutrition and fitness information over the years but just hadn't acted on it. Combining that knowledge with additional research and advice from personal trainers, he set about developing a nutrition and fitness plan that he could follow and sustain over the long haul. One breakthrough was his embrace of portion control and substitution. "I loved chips," he says, "but instead of eating a bag with multiple servings, I would eat from a single-serving bag . . . or I'd grab popcorn instead of chips." And the mayonnaise Jeremiah loved as a kid? He switched to hummus.

It worked. Within six months of starting his new program, he had developed a leaner, stronger body and greater self-confidence. Looking back on his dalliance with diet pills, Jeremiah chuckles, recognizing that a quick fix is never a substitute for lifestyle changes.

MYTH OR TRUTH?

Probiotics promote weight loss.

As discussed in chapter 2, some research shows that people with obesity tend to have a different mix of gut microbes than leaner folks. This has led to the idea that probiotics, which are beneficial bacteria that you can get from supplements and certain foods such as yogurt, may help control weight by altering the mix of microbes (known as the microbiota). While research in rodents supports this notion, human trials have produced mixed results. Some studies have found that probiotics slightly reduce weight, while others show they have no effect or even pack on pounds. One reason for the inconsistency is that trials have used various types of probiotics—there are numerous strains—delivered in different ways (via pills or food) and in different doses. In addition, the studies have been small and in many cases poorly designed. It's therefore unclear which specific probiotics, if any, are effective for weight control. For now, a better approach may be to include plenty of fiber in your diet, which some research suggests can positively affect the microbiota.

Pill Pushers

Through the years, doctors have promoted the use of pills to control weight, often in violation of their ethical obligation to "first do no harm." For example, in the late 19th century, they began prescribing thyroid extract for weight loss under the erroneous theory that thyroid dysfunction was a major cause of obesity. The treatment led to side effects such as heart palpitations, weakness, and nervousness (signs of excess thyroid hormone), which doctors attempted to manage by combining the thyroid extract with arsenic, strychnine, or the heart medicine digitalis. Needless to say, such remedies didn't always work out so well for the recipients.

The 1940s brought rainbow pills, so named because they came in a variety of bright colors. The medications contained combinations of ingredients including thyroid hormones, amphetamines, diuretics, and laxatives, along with barbiturates and other drugs to counter side effects. Sold by manufacturers to doctors, who then dispensed them directly to patients, rainbow pills helped boost the incomes of many physicians.

Though mainstream medicine frowned on the use of these drugs, doctors continued to sell them for several decades, often at pill clinics devoted exclusively to weight loss. Meanwhile, the dangers of amphetamines became increasingly clear, and reports of serious side effects and deaths due to rainbow pills mounted. But the FDA failed to take action. Finally, after a 1968 Senate investigation drew national attention to the pills' dangers, the agency began cracking down on the drugs. By the 1970s, rainbow pills largely disappeared in the US.

Two decades later came another medication craze: fen-phen, a combination of the prescription appetite suppressants fenfluramine (Pondimin) and phentermine. After languishing for years in relative obscurity, the drugs got a huge boost in 1992 when a study showed that taking them together led to an average weight loss of more than 25 pounds over two years, and helped participants keep weight off for nearly four years.

The medications were not approved for long-term use or in combination. But doctors are free to prescribe approved drugs in unapproved ways—a practice called off-label use—and prescribe they did as news spread about the impressive findings.

Physicians working everywhere from private practices to weight-loss centers to universities jumped on the bandwagon and doled out the drugs. Diet-pill clinics—so-called pill mills—sprang up across the country to capitalize on the exploding demand, often by people who wanted to drop just a few pounds. A family practitioner who opened a chain of 18 clinics told the *Wall Street Journal* that his business was raking in $15 million a year. An anesthesiologist owner of 24 clinics boasted to the *Journal*, "You may be talking to the next billionaire!"

By 1996, doctors were writing more than 18 million prescriptions for fen-phen, and millions more for a newly approved version of fenfluramine called Redux, hailed on the cover of one doctor's book as "the most important weight-loss discovery of the century."

But the euphoria soon fizzled when, in 1997, doctors at the Mayo Clinic reported in the *New England Journal of Medicine* that they had detected heart-valve abnormalities in 24 female fen-phen users. Soon the FDA received reports of many more cases, including ones involving Redux. When tests of 291 people taking the drugs showed that one-third had damaged valves, it was the final nail in the coffin. At the FDA's request, the manufacturers pulled fenfluramine and Redux off the market, putting an end to the fen-phen phenomenon. (This side effect was not associated with phentermine, which continues to be sold, as you'll see below.)

In recent years, safety concerns have led to the demise of other weight-loss prescription drugs, including lorcaserin (Belviq), which was withdrawn in 2020 after being linked to cancer, and sibutramine (Meridia), which as previously mentioned was associated with an elevated risk of heart attacks and strokes.

Medications currently on the market (as of this writing) include:

Bupropion-naltrexone (Contrave): Combines an antidepressant and a drug used to treat alcohol and drug dependence. Reduces hunger and controls cravings.

Liraglutide (Saxenda): An injectable drug. Controls appetite by mimicking a hormone that signals to the brain you're full.

Semaglutide (Wegovy): Works in a similar way to liraglutide. Both belong to the same class of medications and are also used to treat type 2 diabetes.

Orlistat (Xenical): Also sold over the counter as Alli, in a lower dose. Blocks the absorption of fat.

Phentermine-topiramate (Qsymia): The phen in fen-phen is now paired up with an antiseizure medication. The combo suppresses appetite, but the exact mechanism isn't fully understood.

These medications, which are intended only for people who have obesity or who are overweight and have conditions such as diabetes, have generally been shown in trials to shave off roughly 5 to 20 more pounds over 12 months (depending on the drug) than diet and lifestyle counseling. Initial studies of Wegovy, the most recently approved medication, suggest it may be more effective. People taking the drugs are more likely to lose at least 5 percent of their weight and keep lost pounds off.

But these benefits come with a price: a long list of potential side effects. They vary from one drug to another, but the most common include gastrointestinal problems such as nausea, diarrhea, constipation, and vomiting, as well as headaches, dry mouth, altered taste perception, and tingling of the skin. The high frequency of side effects has led to dropout rates of up to 45 percent in studies.

So, while these drugs can be helpful in some cases, they're no picnic—and no panacea. People taking them still need to make diet and lifestyle changes to achieve long-term success. Recognizing these limitations, many physicians are hesitant to prescribe the drugs. By one estimate, less than 3 percent of people with obesity take them.

Some in the medical community see this as a problem—that an effective weight-control tool is being underused. Perhaps. Or maybe it's a sign that doctors have learned the lessons from the past 100-plus years about the perils of irrational exuberance when it comes to weight-loss drugs. With more in the research pipeline (some of which are already being hyped as "game changers"), we can only hope.

MYTH OR TRUTH?

Hormone treatments are a good way to control weight.

It's true that levels of certain hormones affect weight and body composition. In women, for example, the drop in estrogen associated with menopause can lead to increased abdominal fat. In men, declining testosterone levels, which occur with age, may have the same effect. And weight gain is one of the symptoms of hypothyroidism—a condition in which the thyroid gland doesn't produce enough hormone. But taking hormones, which may be appropriate for boosting levels that are truly low or reducing menopausal symptoms, is unacceptably risky as a weight-control strategy. A "black box" warning on thyroid hormone, for instance, states that it's not for weight loss because too much of the hormone can lead to "serious or even life threatening" effects. Estrogen replacement therapy can raise women's risk of dementia, heart attacks, and strokes, and some research has linked testosterone therapy to cardio-vascular problems.

Despite claims to the contrary, there's no proof that "bioidentical" hormones from compounding pharmacies are safer or better options. Nor is there solid evidence that nat-ural ingredients in supplements can "rebalance" hormones. Instead, focus on lifestyle measures like a healthful diet, reg-ular exercise (including resistance training), adequate sleep, and stress management. (For more on these, see chapter 8.)

The Wild, Wild West

At a congressional hearing in 2014, senators castigated Dr. Oz for repeatedly plugging weight-loss supplements on his show with words like "magic" and "miracle."

"I don't get why you need to say this stuff," said Senator Claire McCaskill, "because you know it's not true."

The lawmakers were right to point out that Oz, whose effusive praise for questionable compounds like green cof-fee extract, raspberry ketone, and *Garcinia cambogia* helped fuel their popularity, has been part of the problem when it comes to supplements. His defense—that he personally believes in the products and should be able to use what he called "flowery" language—was less than satisfying.

But if elected leaders want to know where the blame ultimately lies, they should look in the mirror. DSHEA, the law passed by Congress governing the regulation of supple-ments, has resulted in a Wild West of weight-loss pills where the sheriffs are stripped of their authority. Lawmakers' failure to fix the problem they created leaves us vulnerable to modern-day snake-oil peddlers and undermines our efforts at weight control.

One way this plays out is that we waste lots of money on useless remedies—funds that could be spent on more effective measures like healthful foods, nutrition counseling, or behavioral therapy for weight loss.

In addition, we may jeopardize our health. In a study of visits to hospital emergency departments due to supplement side effects, weight-loss products were the most common culprits among women. For both male and female weight-loss supplement users, the most frequent symptoms were cardiac-related issues such as chest pain and heart palpitations. In fact, the hospitals tied such effects more often to weight-loss supplements than to prescription stimulants.

What we know about side effects, which can be caused by "natural" ingredients found on the label or adulterants such as prescription drugs that aren't listed, is likely just the tip of the iceberg. Supplement makers aren't required to test for safety, and the FDA's voluntary system for reporting adverse events from supplements, known as CAERS, is flawed and woefully underutilized.

When we have inadequate information about potential harms, we can't balance risks against benefits to make rational judgments about a supplement. As a result, we may be more likely to fall prey to marketing come-ons and to sabotage our health while doing little or nothing to help our weight.

A less obvious way that supplements may lead us astray is by weakening our dietary self-control. Evidence for this comes from a study involving women who wanted to lose weight. Researchers randomized them to receive either a weight-loss supplement (which was actually a placebo) or an actual placebo (which the subjects were told was inert).

After taking the pills, they had a buffet lunch where their food consumption was secretly monitored. Participants who believed they had swallowed a weight-loss pill helped themselves to more food and were more apt to choose unhealthy items like cookies, fries, and soda than those who thought they had taken a placebo.

It's a phenomenon akin to what we see with foods that have "health halos," which can lead people to mistakenly believe that they have greater license to indulge. In the same way, supplements may make some users feel more entitled to eat whatever they want because they think they're addressing their weight by popping a pill. That's especially true if they believe a product has the power to melt away pounds regardless of diet.

If you want to try a supplement for weight loss, don't expect too much, and remember that you still need to pay attention to what you eat. If you're taking medications or receiving medical care, talk to a health-care provider or pharmacist to make sure the supplement doesn't interfere with your treatment.

If you're a candidate for prescription weight-loss medications and are considering them, it's important to carefully assess risks and benefits with your provider. While the drugs can provide a leg up for certain people, they too are not a replacement for a healthy diet and other weight-control measures.

From DNP to DMAA, fen-phen to forskolin, and amphetamines to orlistat, the quest for a solution in a bottle has been a constant theme in weight-loss history since the 19th century. Despite the steady stream of scams, false promises, and deadly consequences, many of us today continue to hold out hope that a pill or potion of some sort can come to our rescue. Perhaps medical science will eventually fulfill that wish with a weight-loss medication that's both highly safe and highly effective. But for now, we're better off putting our faith in diet and lifestyle measures—a truth that for many people is a hard pill to swallow.

What to Do

- ⊃ View claims for weight-loss supplements with skepticism, and remember that the products aren't risk-free.

- ⊃ If you want to try a supplement, buy from a reputable seller. Look for products that list the amount of every major ingredient. Check whether the supplement has been tested by Consumerlab.com or Labdoor.com, both of which analyze supplements to see whether they contain what's on the label as well as any impurities, pharmaceuticals, or other undisclosed ingredients.

- ⊃ If your weight and health status qualify you for prescription weight-loss medications, discuss the pros and cons with a health-care provider

Chapter 7

UNREAL IDEAL

If you happen to be visiting Columbus, Ohio, and feel an urge to weigh yourself, Christopher Steele likely has a scale you can use. Actually, 150 of them. Just be sure to bring a penny.

Steele owns the nation's premier collection of penny scales. The machines, which first appeared in the US in the 1880s, eventually became ubiquitous, popping up everywhere from banks and train stations to drugstores and movie theaters. For many years, these public scales were the only way that most people could check their weight unless they visited a doctor's office.

In contrast to the sense of dread that weighing ourselves often elicits today, stepping onto a penny scale could be fun and entertaining thanks to manufacturers' gimmicks. Customers might get their fortunes, play games of chance (which included guessing their own weight), or receive printed tickets with collectible pictures of movie stars. Some scales could talk, announcing the person's weight aloud—a feature that most of us now would greet with horror.

There were also scales that displayed health messages about weight. For example, one sign from Steele's collection proclaims, "Your waistline is your healthline. Weigh yourself once a day." Another, which shows a tombstone, offers up this ditty: "Shed a tear for kareless Kate. She forgot to watch her weight."

At their peak in the 1930s, the scales brought in 10 billion pennies annually ($100 million if you do the math), according to Steele. But after World War II, the machines went the way of the horse and buggy because of the increased popularity of bathroom scales, which allowed people to weigh themselves unclothed in the privacy of their own homes.

Today's home scales come with high-tech features including Bluetooth capability and apps that let you track readings through your cell phone, fitness tracker, smart watch, or smart speaker (a modern-day—and less embarrassing—version of the talking penny scale). Some scales can distinguish among multiple users and automatically recognize who you are when you step on. What's more, many also provide readings on other metrics, including body fat, bone mass, metabolic rate, "body age," and heart rate—pretty much everything except your shoe size and IQ.

The technology we use to weigh ourselves, like that in so many other areas of our lives, has advanced tremendously. But how we interpret the readings has not. To determine what we're supposed to weigh, doctors and weight-loss experts frequently rely on tools that are no more sophisticated than the simplistic weight charts posted on penny scales 100 years ago. In some cases, modern-day weight metrics cause undue alarm about our health, while in others they provide false assurances by labeling those who are metabolically unhealthy as "normal."

What's more, popular culture sets standards regarding body size that are impossible for most of us to meet. This skewed view of "ideal" often leads to unrealistic expectations about what we should weigh, along with disappointment and self-blame when we fail to reach unattainable goals. It may also prompt us to give the number on the scale too much weight.

Christopher Steele says he'd like to see a return of scales in public places. If that ever occurred, perhaps the old slogans could be replaced with a new one about interpreting the readings: "Proceed with Caution."

Shifting Standards

The concept of ideal weight originated with the life insurance industry, which beginning in the early 20th century found that policyholders past their early to mid-30s with above-average weights had higher mortality rates. (In younger people, being underweight correlated with an elevated death rate because of increased susceptibility to tuberculosis.)

Initially, insurance companies created height and weight tables that showed average weights, but eventually the standard changed to *ideal* weights—those at which mortality rates were lowest. The notion that everyone should aim for a particular target really took off in the early 1940s, when Metropolitan Life published ideal ranges for adults based on gender, height, and frame size. The ideal weight for a medium-framed woman standing 5 feet, 4 inches was 124 to 132. For a medium-framed man who was 5 feet, 9 inches tall, it was 149 to 160.

Aside from specifying that the ranges applied to people 25 and older, the Metropolitan Life tables did not take age into account. Thus, a 75-year-old was supposed to weigh the same as a 25-year-old. Similarly, there was no consideration of race or ethnicity. Though the actuarial data upon which the tables were based came from predominantly white policyholders, the recommended weights were supposed to apply to everyone. What's more, the definitions of small, medium, and large frame sizes were ambiguous.

Nevertheless, the medical profession embraced the insurance tables, as did the general public. Updated over the years, they remained for decades the definitive guide to what people should weigh.

But not everyone was on board. Among the critics was Ancel Keys—the same researcher who, as mentioned in chapter 1, linked saturated fat to heart disease. In a 1972 study using data collected from more than 7,400 men, Keys analyzed several mathematical formulas for indicating body fatness and concluded the winner to be what he dubbed the body mass index. It was a new name for an old concept.

Originally called the Quetelet index, it was developed by Belgian mathematician Adolphe Quetelet in 1832. Seeking to define characteristics of the "average" man, Quetelet gathered data on weights and heights, and came up with a ratio between the two (weight/height^2) to fit the distribution under a bell-shaped curve.

Quetelet was a polymath whose research spanned an array of fields including astronomy, sociology, and criminology. But medicine was not among them. He was not a physician, and his index was never intended as a way to assess weight or health in individuals. It was a statistical tool for describing populations.

Yet, thanks to the resurrection and rebranding of Quetelet's work by Keys, body mass index, or BMI, soon became the standard yardstick for categorizing people according to weight. In a 1985 report on obesity by a panel of experts, the NIH officially recommended that doctors use BMI to evaluate patients, calling it "a simple measurement highly correlated with other estimates of fatness."

I'm not so sure about the "simple" part. BMI is calculated by dividing your weight in kilograms by your height in meters squared. Alternatively, you can divide your weight in pounds by height in inches squared and multiply that amount by 703. Got that?

What *is* simple is that BMI involves just two measurements—height and weight—and there are plenty of charts and online calculators that do the math for you. Interpreting the results is seemingly straightforward as well. A BMI of 18.5 to 24.9 is considered normal. Twenty-five to 29.9 means you're overweight, and 30 or higher indicates obesity.

In fact, these tidy cutoffs are fairly arbitrary, and small shifts can make a big difference in how people are classified. In 1998, when the NIH moved the dividing line between normal and overweight slightly downward to make the cutoffs consistent with those of the World Health Organization, 29 million Americans who had been classified as normal suddenly became overweight without gaining a pound.

Defective Metric

The arbitrariness of BMI categories is just one of the tool's shortcomings. Despite its widespread use by everyone from doctors to dietitians to fitness instructors, BMI has a number of drawbacks that can mislead us about our weight and health.

BMI is intended to identify people who are carrying excess fat, which is what can lead to health problems. But the metric doesn't distinguish between fat and the other components of weight, including muscle and bone. As a result, someone who's muscular and athletic can have a high BMI and be labeled "obese" even though their body fat is relatively low.

Conversely, people who have low muscle mass but a relatively large amount of internal fat may fall in the "normal" range. In fact, research suggests that BMI misses half of those with excess fat. This may be especially relevant for older folks because we tend to gain fat and lose muscle as we age, even if our weight doesn't change. Yet, like the height and weight charts it eventually replaced, BMI doesn't take age into account.

The same goes for race. BMI was derived from measurements in white Europeans and has universal cutoffs between weight categories, with no adjustments for different populations. This can lead to skewed results for Black people, who on average have heavier bones and greater muscle mass than Caucasians. Consequently their BMI readings are more likely to overestimate fatness. On the other hand, Asians tend to have body builds that cause BMI to underestimate body fat.

Yet another problem is that BMI doesn't reveal where fat is located, which is important. As discussed previously, visceral fat—the type deep in the abdomen and indicated by a large waist—is associated with a greater risk of heart disease, diabetes, and other health problems. In contrast to an "apple" shape due to excess abdominal fat, having a "pear" shape—meaning fat concentrated mainly around the hips, thighs, or butt—isn't linked to these risks. While women tend to have more body fat than men, they're less likely to carry it in their abdomens—an important difference that BMI doesn't capture.

Given all these limitations, it's no surprise that BMI isn't always a good indicator of health status. In a study involving data from more than 40,000 adults, researchers classified participants' metabolic health based on measures including blood pressure, cholesterol, insulin resistance, and C-reactive protein (a measure of inflammation). Nearly half of people labeled as overweight by BMI turned out to be metabolically healthy, as did 29 percent who fell in the "obese" range. At the same time, nearly one-third of those in the "normal" weight category were metabolically *unhealthy.* The researchers estimated that relying mainly on BMI would misclassify the metabolic health of nearly 75 million Americans.

Granted, the metabolic measurements in this cross-sectional study were snapshots that don't indicate outcomes years or decades later. Some research that has followed subjects over time suggests that metabolically healthy people deemed obese according to BMI are more likely than healthy, normal-weight individuals to eventually develop cardiovascular disease and diabetes.

Nevertheless, the fact remains that BMI is a crude instrument from the 1800s that too often fails to accurately measure what it's supposed to. The inadequacies of BMI are no secret—there are countless studies documenting its deficiencies—yet many in the weight-loss industry continue to embrace it. One reason is inertia; old habits die hard. Another is that other methods involve measurements that are less convenient to obtain than height and weight.

One such alternative is waist size. Studies show that even among people whose BMI falls in the normal range, having a larger waist is associated with a greater risk of premature death. But it's harder to measure waist circumference accurately than height and weight. Readings can vary depending on exactly where the tape measure is placed— and whether you're able to resist the temptation to suck in your stomach. When you last ate can also have an effect.

In addition, there's disagreement about where the cutoffs should lie. While many health authorities including the NIH recommend a waist circumference of no more than 40 inches in men and 35 inches in nonpregnant women, others argue that these thresholds aren't optimal for all populations and should be adjusted for different ethnic and racial groups.

Sometimes both waist size and hip circumference are measured to calculate a waist-to-hip ratio. In other cases, a waist-to-height ratio is used. Still other tools combine waist circumference with BMI. Whether adding waist size to other measurements is superior to using waist size alone, and if so, which ones are best, remains a matter of debate.

Therein lies perhaps the biggest reason that BMI continues its undeserved reign as king of body-fat measurements: there's no agreed-upon contender to dethrone it. As physician and author Sylvia Karasu writes, "Despite all the progress we have made in science since Quetelet's 19th century index, we are still far away from being able to measure our body's fat conveniently and accurately."

MYTH OR TRUTH?

Body-fat scales are accurate.

Scales that measure body fat, which you can buy for home use or find in gyms, rely on a technology known as bioelectrical impedance analysis, or BIA. When you step onto the scale, it sends a small, imperceptible electric current through your body. Fat causes more resistance (impedance) than muscle, so the greater the resistance, the greater the body fat. The scales put this information into a formula, along with data that users enter, such as height, age, and gender, to calculate the percentage of body fat. But this is only an estimate, and it's frequently off. A test of six home scales by Consumer Reports found that all were inaccurate, with error rates ranging from 21 to 34 percent. For some subjects the readings were too low, and for others too high. A number of factors can affect results, including body shape, hydration status, and recent exercise activity. There are also handheld BIA devices, which aren't any more accurate.

As for alternatives, skin-pinch tests, which use calipers to measure skinfold thickness, can also be error prone because their accuracy depends on the tester's skill. More reliable options include underwater weighing and DEXA scans, which involve low-energy X-rays like those used to measure bone density. But these methods are less convenient than BIA scales and skin-pinch tests.

Do I Look Fat?

Of course, BMI and other measurements aren't the only benchmarks for judging whether we're the "right" weight. Societal norms play an important role as well.

Before the 20th century, the ideal female body, as depicted in sculpture and paintings, was full-figured. But that changed with the emergence of the tall, narrow-waisted Gibson Girl in the 1890s. For two decades, she was the wildly popular embodiment of the feminine ideal, appearing in magazines and newspapers, and on calendars and other merchandise. Women strove to emulate her. Never mind that this woman didn't really exist. She was a drawing that sprang from the imagination of a man, artist Charles Dana Gibson.

The Roaring '20s brought the flapper, the slim, corset-free woman who rebelled against Victorian constraints. Curves were out, and an adolescent—almost boyish—body was in. To fit into the short, revealing dresses of the era, women often turned to dieting. Capitalizing on the trend, makers of diet-related products used mass advertising— then a new phenomenon—to hawk their offerings, further fueling demand as well as the new thin ideal. These advertisements, writes Laura Fraser in her book *Losing It*, "made women feel humiliated that they weren't as slim as the beautiful women in [the] illustrations."

In the decades that followed, Hollywood stars came to play a powerful role in shaping the ideal as well. Early stirrings of this influence were evident in a 1932 article in the *New Movie Magazine*. Titled "How the Stars Keep Slim and Trim," it reported that actress Dorothy Jordan did a "daily check against dangerous curves" to make sure that her measurements stayed below 33-24½-36 and her weight didn't exceed 108 pounds. The story, which described Jordan's diet and exercise routine, showed the super-skinny young woman clad in a short skirt, standing on a penny scale.

In the 1950s, sex symbols like Marilyn Monroe briefly brought fuller bodies back in vogue. With a waist of 22 inches, though, she was hardly plump. The introduction of Barbie in 1959 offered young girls an even-less-attainable ideal: If scaled to the size of a real person standing 5 feet, 9 inches, she would weigh in at 110 pounds and have an 18-inch waist. Likewise, the emaciated model Twiggy, who exploded onto the scene in the 1960s, took extreme thinness to new heights, a trend that has continued among models and celebrities.

Analyzing the body sizes of fashion models, *Playboy* Playmates of the Year, and Miss America pageant winners over the course of the 20th century, researchers found that the women's BMIs steadily declined. In the 1920s, for example, Miss America winners had BMIs between 20 and 25, putting them in the normal range. By the 1970s, however, most were falling into the "underweight" category.

Facing criticism for promoting an unhealthy body image with rail-thin models, the fashion industry has begun to showcase a greater diversity of body types in recent years. Likewise, Barbie now comes in several shapes, and more celebrities emphasize health over weight when promoting their regimens.

Nevertheless, thin is still very much in. For evidence, look no further than the covers of women's magazines, including those related to health and fitness, which typically feature models that one analysis concluded are often "conspicuously thin."

On social media, the thin ideal is just as evident, and exposure to it is potentially far greater because of the sheer volume of images available. Young women who spend hours a day scrolling through feeds of celebrities like Kendall Jenner or Hailey Bieber are likely to see far more photos of slender bodies than they would viewing traditional media.

When fitness blogger and YouTube star Cassey Ho analyzed the physical attributes of the 100 most-followed females on Instagram, she found that nearly 90 percent had flat stomachs. The most common body type was hourglass, followed by thin and straight. Only five of the 100 influencers were plus size; none of the top 10 were. So much for body diversity.

The fact that women know these images are often Photoshopped doesn't necessarily diminish their influence. Research suggests that the more time young women spend on social media, especially viewing appearance-related content, the more likely they are to internalize the thin body ideal.

While there's less research on the effects of media among middle-aged and older women, studies suggest that this ideal—whether it comes from social media, TV, movies, magazines, or advertising—influences how women of all ages perceive their own bodies and weight status.

In men, exposure to the media's depiction of the "ideal" male physique—typically lean with well-defined muscles—may similarly affect how some see themselves. But generally, the impact on men appears to be less pronounced than that of the female ideal on women.

While the effects of these body ideals vary from person to person, it's indisputable that societal standards, as shaped and reflected by various forms of media, can influence how we think we should look and what we think we should weigh.

Our own ideas and experiences often play a role as well. Perhaps our ideal is what we weighed in college or our lowest weight ever or the weight of a friend or family member. Maybe it's a weight we've always dreamed of achieving or simply a number that sounds good—say, 20 or 50 or 100 pounds lighter.

Whatever the case, if we rely on dreams and wishes or societal norms or BMI charts to determine our ideal weight, we can be led astray. The "right" weight, it turns out, depends on what's healthy, reasonable, and sustainable for you—goals you can't achieve by picking a number on a scale or chart, or trying to emulate an airbrushed Instagram image.

Diana's Journey

As a kid, Diana was tall and developed early. Whenever she looked in the mirror, she says she always thought she "looked fat," even though she now sees from old photos that she wasn't overweight. Diana started dieting in the fourth grade, and throughout her adolescence turned to extreme exercise and restrictive diets to control her weight.

The distorted body image persisted in college, where Diana became known as "the cereal girl" because that's all she ate in order to keep her weight down. When she started working at a restaurant after college, she began eating and drinking more, which led to weight gain. Trying one diet after another, which always left her feeling deprived, she says, "I dieted myself fatter and fatter."

Diana's weight ballooned to the point that she could not fit into a restaurant booth. At 250 pounds, she decided to try something different, this time following a less-restrictive approach to eating that she could sustain. Over the course of a year, she dropped 100 pounds.

To maintain the weight loss, she stepped up her exercise, eventually running a 31-mile ultramarathon. The exercise became excessive, causing her to lose more weight and putting her health in jeopardy. This led her to the realization that "being my smallest is not better." Listening to her body, Diana has allowed herself to regain some weight, and as a result, she says she's now healthier.

Despite her major weight loss, she continues to struggle with the urge to be as thin as possible, a lifelong quest that she says has hurt her self-esteem. Diana admits there's still a voice in her head telling her, "You could be smaller if you tried." She answers by reminding herself that good health, not the scale, is what defines "ideal" weight.

MYTH OR TRUTH?

Weight status is "contagious."

The notion that obesity can spread like a virus from person to person has, well, spread in recent years. And there's evidence to back it up. For example, a study of 12,000 people found that someone's chances of becoming obese increased if a friend became obese. To a lesser extent, the same was true if a sibling or spouse became obese. Your community may play a role as well. In research involving military families, those assigned to live at installations in US counties with higher obesity rates were more prone to be obese than those living in counties with lower obesity rates.

This "social contagion," as researchers call it, also applies to weight loss: We're more likely to lose weight, or at least attempt to, if friends or spouses are doing so. One possible explanation is that we tend to mirror the behaviors of people around us, including habits related to eating and weight. Another is that our social network helps shape what's considered a "normal" weight. If friends and family members are thinner than we are, we may feel more pressure to lose weight than if we're surrounded by people who are heavy. The upshot is that while the research as a whole doesn't prove cause and effect, it does suggest that being around others who are at, or moving toward, a healthy weight may be beneficial.

Great Expectations

Wherever they come from, misguided beliefs about ideal weight can lead to unrealistic expectations about weight loss. In a widely cited study, 60 obese women beginning a weight-loss program were asked to name their "dream" weight, "happy" weight, "acceptable" weight, and "disappointed" weight. On average, reaching dream and happy weights would require them to lose more than 30 percent of their body weight—a result far exceeding what most people are able to achieve unless they undergo bariatric surgery. And indeed in this study, only 9 percent of participants reached their happy weight after a year, and none got down to their dream weight. What's more, nearly half failed to end up at even their disappointed weight—even though they lost an impressive 36 pounds on average.

Other studies have also found that people's desired weights tend to be unrealistic. Overall, research shows that expectations tend to be highest in women and in people who are younger and the most overweight.

In some cases, doctors may contribute to these inflated hopes, or at least do nothing to dispel them. In a survey of primary care physicians, their definitions of "dream" and "happy" outcomes for patients were just as over the top as laypeople's notions. Further, nearly one-third of the doctors reported that they would consider losing between 5 and 10 percent of body weight to be disappointing, even though this result is realistic for weight-reduction programs and is linked to health benefits.

For some people, lofty expectations can be motivating, especially at first. And certainly optimism and a belief in our own ability to succeed (what psychologists call self-efficacy) are necessary to accomplish anything that's challenging, like weight loss. But expecting too much may derail our efforts.

For example, in an Italian study of nearly 1,800 people enrolled in a weight-loss program, those with the highest expectations were more likely to have dropped out by the 12-month mark. One possible explanation is a phenomenon known as the *false-hope syndrome*: the notion that unrealistic expectations set us up for failure, disappointment, and a sense of defeat.

Now, not all studies show that false hope leads people over time to get discouraged and abandon weight-loss efforts. It's possible, for example, that some people lower their expectations when reality sets in, and they end up feeling satisfied with more modest outcomes.

But it stands to reason that many of us may become disillusioned and demoralized when we get results that are far short of what we had hoped for. This disappointment may not only dampen or destroy our motivation but also contribute to self-blame and all the harmful effects associated with it.

What's more, having an unattainable ideal weight may contribute in some people to disordered eating and yo-yo dieting, also known as weight cycling. In a study of middle-aged people, higher expectations of thinness were associated with more weight cycling, including episodes of losing and regaining at least 20 pounds, regardless of gender or BMI. Though research overall is inconclusive about the health risks of weight cycling, some studies have linked it to effects including greater fat accumulation and an increased risk of diabetes.

Diet-plan pushers would have us believe that by following their regimens we all can be as slim and chiseled as the bodies shown in their ads. Unfortunately, that's not the case. A weight that's attainable for you may not be attainable for me, or vice versa. It all depends on factors such as starting weight, gender, and genetics. Age plays a role as well; changes in muscle mass, hormones, and metabolism make it harder to lose weight as we get older.

Regardless of what weight we might hope and believe is attainable, our bodies often have a different idea. One theory of weight regulation is that we all have a genetically influenced range where the body tries mightily to remain— its own "ideal" weight. When we severely restrict calories or fall below our range, our bodies fight back. As discussed in chapter 2, this resistance comes in several forms, including increased hunger and decreased metabolism, which serve to drive our weight back up in a misdirected effort to protect us from starvation.

For most of us, it's not too hard to push this range upward. When we pack on pounds, the body often considers the higher weight its new ideal and stays there (though for some people, the body does fight back, making it hard for them to keep extra weight on). Resetting the range downward is typically much tougher, and there's no definitive science on how to do so.

Remaining under your body's ideal range is possible, but it's an uphill struggle that can make life difficult. As Traci Mann advises in her book *Secrets from the Eating Lab*, "Unless you want to battle evolution, biology, and psychology and be hungry every single day of your life, I wouldn't suggest trying to live below your set range."

Instead, Mann advises figuring out where your body wants to be and staying at the low end of that range—in short, adjusting the ideal weight in your mind to match the one in your body.

MYTH OR TRUTH?

Weighing yourself every day increases weight loss.

Some diet plans and weight-loss experts recommend frequent weighing, and science backs them up—but with some important caveats. A review of 19 trials concluded that overweight people who step on the scale frequently—ideally every day—lose more weight and regain less than those who don't. For some people, carefully tracking weight yields feedback to keep them accountable, and seeing favorable trends provides motivation to continue. For others, though, frequent weighing can have negative psychological effects, including stress and reduced self-esteem. In some cases, it may also contribute to unhealthy eating behaviors.

Keep in mind that readings can be deceiving. Daily fluctuations are often due to factors such as changes in body water or hormones. And the typical scale doesn't reveal anything about the proportions of fat and muscle. Losing a pound of fat and gaining a pound of muscle, for example, registers as no change. Most important, weight is just one way among several to gauge success, including how healthy you are, how your clothes fit, and how you feel. If you can keep your readings in perspective and not obsess over them, frequent weighing may be beneficial. Otherwise, it's best to use the scale more sparingly.

When Positivity Turns Negative

One response to society's thin ideal is the body positivity movement, which promotes the idea that bodies come in all shapes and sizes, and that people shouldn't base their self-worth on what they look like or what their number on the scale happens to be. As discussed previously, weight stigma inflicts harm in a number of ways, ranging from bias and discrimination to self-blame and low self-esteem. The movement's efforts to combat this stigma, along with the misguided ideas of diet culture that contribute to it, should be applauded.

But body positivity isn't so positive when it downplays or denies the health risks of obesity, as is sometimes the case. The same goes when it discourages people, whether explicitly or implicitly, from wanting to lose weight to improve their health. In fact, research shows that heavy people who lose even relatively modest amounts of weight may experience a number of benefits, including a lower risk of diabetes and improvements in blood pressure, cholesterol, sleep apnea, and arthritis of the knee. They also report improved quality of life.

Advocates of body positivity who claim that weight is not connected to health are just as guilty of spreading misinformation as those on the other side who claim that we all can become thin if we diet and exercise enough. In a *New York Times* essay titled "The Problem with Body Positivity," author Kelly deVos, a self-described "fat woman" who had bought into the idea that her size didn't pose a risk, writes about coming to terms with the health realities of excess weight after learning she has diabetes. Challenging the taboo against weight loss among some body positivity proponents, she concludes: "Loving yourself and desiring to change yourself are two sentiments that should be able to peacefully coexist."

The antidote to the thin ideal isn't—or shouldn't be—complete indifference to weight. Instead, we should pay attention to our weight. But we should also see it for what it is: just one barometer of our well-being that must be considered in the context of other indicators, such as diet quality, physical activity level, metabolic health, emotional health, and functional abilities.

Think of it this way: When it comes to your *financial* well-being, your income certainly matters. But so do other things like how much you spend on food and housing, how much you save, and how much you splurge.

The "right" income for you depends on these other factors, and odds are it won't match the "ideal" of winning the lottery or earning what LeBron James does. The same goes for weight. What's right for you depends largely on other measures of well-being. And it may fall well short of some unrealistic ideal you've been led to embrace.

Put another way, the weight to aim for is what Drs. Yoni Freedhoff and Arya Sharma call your "best" weight, which they define as the weight people are able to achieve "while living the healthiest lifestyle they can truly enjoy." This may not be your lowest weight ever or one you get from a BMI calculator or see on a magazine cover. Instead it's a weight that, for you, is attainable and sustainable while enhancing your health and well-being.

Whatever that number happens to be—and it may very well change throughout your life—it shouldn't dictate your self-worth. Imagine a relationship with the scale in which your weight doesn't define who you are but does provide one piece of data to help you lead a healthier life. Now, that's what I call ideal.

What to Do

➲ Shoot for a weight that you can realistically achieve and maintain. Remember that losing just 5 to 10 percent of your body weight can yield health benefits.

➲ Don't put too much stock in your BMI reading. Instead, pay attention to your waist size and other indicators of metabolic health, including blood pressure, cholesterol, and blood sugar.

➲ Weigh yourself regularly if you find it helpful. But don't obsess over the number on the scale.

Chapter 8

WHAT WORKS

My job involves keeping up with the latest health trends, and one way I do that is to scan publications while I'm in line in the supermarket checkout aisle. (Okay, I admit I sometimes also look at articles about farmers in Kansas being abducted by aliens.)

When it comes to stories about weight loss, I've noticed one word that appears over and over in headlines: *secrets.* You can read about "Best Diet Secrets," "One-Minute Summer Weight Loss Secrets," "Weight Loss Secrets Only Nutritionists Know," and of course "Stars' Secrets."

Another word these publications seem to love is *shortcut.* Articles promise to reveal "Shortcuts to Lasting Weight Loss," "Weight Loss Shortcuts That Actually Work," and the "#1 Weight Loss Shortcut."

If there were a contest for fake news, these headlines would definitely deserve a prize.

Contrary to what we often hear, there are in fact no secrets or shortcuts to weight loss. For evidence of this unfortunate reality, consider a study that compared 14 popular diet plans. Analyzing trials involving a total of more than 20,000 participants, the research found that during the first six months all the diets led to weight loss—some a bit more than others—but by 12 months the differences in outcomes were negligible. As an accompanying editorial put it, there's "a plethora of choice but no clear winner."

That conclusion is further supported by studies from the National Weight Control Registry (NWCR), which, as mentioned in chapter 3, tracks people who have lost at least 30 pounds and kept it off long term. One of the takeaways from research on the more than 10,000 participants is this: There's no one solution that explains their success. To reach their mutual destination, these folks have followed different paths that include various combinations of strategies. The key to long-term weight control, according to researchers studying the participants, is "finding a set of behaviors that works for each individual and maintaining these behaviors over time"—hardly an earth-shattering "secret."

Though there's no one-size-fits-all solution, there *are* basic principles grounded in science that can help with long-term weight control, which typically requires a multipronged attack. Notice that I said "principles" and not "rules." These aren't strict dos and don'ts. Instead, they're guidelines to apply in a way that works for you.

They include healthful eating, a healthy lifestyle, self-monitoring, planning for challenges, and professional assistance. Here's what each entails and how it can help.

Go the Whole Way

Whether you choose keto, paleo, Atkins, Optifast, or something else, a diet may very well lead to weight loss in the short run. But keeping the weight off requires shifting from a mindset of "dieting"—which implies something that's temporary and demands self-deprivation—to developing eating habits you can sustain for life.

It turns out that the eating pattern that's best for your health—a plant-based diet emphasizing whole foods and minimizing highly processed foods—is also good for your weight. This way of eating isn't complicated or overly restrictive. As previously discussed, it includes broad categories such as vegetables, fruits, whole grains, beans, nuts, and seeds, along with seafood and lean poultry, all of which lend themselves to lots of choices.

One possible reason that such foods help with weight is that many of them (with the notable exceptions of nuts and seeds) tend to be low in energy density, meaning that they contain fewer calories per ounce because they're relatively high in water, fiber, or both. Essentially, they give you more bang for your calorie buck, allowing you to fill up on fewer calories.

According to research, we tend to eat roughly the same volume of food each day. If we can maintain that volume, we don't feel deprived, even when we cut calories via lower energy density. Evidence for this comes from a study in which researchers borrowed a trick from parents of picky eaters: They sneaked pureed vegetables into entrées, which decreased the energy density of the food. Subjects reported feeling just as full from these "watered-down" dishes as they did from versions with higher energy densities.

A number of studies suggest that lowering energy density can be effective for weight control. For instance, a trial involving 132 overweight subjects found that after shedding pounds, those assigned to a low-energy-density eating plan were more successful than the control group at maintaining their weight loss during the three-year follow-up. Likewise, a study that tracked women for six years showed that low-energy-density eaters gained less weight than those whose diets were higher in energy density.

Though research is mixed about the effects of protein on weight management, many people find that including it in every meal, with foods such as plain yogurt, beans, eggs, fish, and skinless poultry, is another way to keep hunger at bay.

On the flip side are choices like chips, candy, cookies, and white bread, which are less likely to fill us up than whole foods. One possible explanation is that these highly processed foods usually have less fiber and bulk. Another is that we tend to eat them more quickly. It can take up to 20 minutes for our brains to get the message that we're full, so the alert may not arrive until after we've devoured that bag of Doritos.

It's also easy to overdo it on juice, soda, and other caloric beverages. Though these are low in energy density because they're liquids, research suggests that drinking your calories is usually less filling than eating them.

Minimizing hunger is essential for any eating plan to be sustainable. And so is the ability to eat foods that you enjoy. As mentioned in chapter 1, completely banning specific foods or entire categories isn't a realistic long-term strategy, and it can make matters worse by ramping up cravings and leading to binge eating. So if you want cake, doughnuts, hot dogs, fast-food fries, or other highly processed foods, that's okay. The key is to make them occasional treats, in limited portions, instead of regular staples.

Getting to that point takes time, so be patient and start with small changes. If you eat a candy bar every day, for example, cut back to every other day and then gradually drop back the frequency from there, trying more healthful options like fruit as a substitute. As your new eating habits become more ingrained, you'll likely find it easier to resist the temptation to indulge in such foods.

Because a whole-food approach to eating allows lots of leeway regarding food choices, trial and error may be necessary to figure out what works best for you. You can include some red meat, no animal foods at all, or something in between. You can incorporate dairy products or not. You can vary the proportions of carbohydrates, fats, and protein depending on your preferences.

This flexibility puts a greater burden on you to figure things out initially. But the effort will pay off in the long run by allowing you to tailor an eating plan that you can stick with. Most important, regardless of your weight, you'll be eating in a way that helps protect your health.

Move, Sleep, and De-stress

Just as a healthful diet contributes to weight control, so does a healthy lifestyle, starting with exercise. As discussed in chapter 3, while exercise is overrated as a way to lose weight, it's important for preventing weight gain. A review of studies from weight-control registries in five countries, including the NWCR in the US, showed physical activity to be consistently associated with better weight-loss maintenance.

Aim to do at least 30 minutes of aerobic activity on most days. It's fine to break it into smaller chunks, and the workouts don't need to be punishing. You can walk, hike, bike, swim, dance, attend a class, or do whatever suits you, as long as it's moderately intense. As with healthy eating, there are lots of choices, and it's crucial to pick activities you enjoy (or at least don't hate) so you'll keep doing them.

In addition, try to do resistance training at least twice a week. Though this type of exercise often gets short shrift, it's an essential part of a well-rounded workout plan for everyone—not just athletes and bodybuilders. And you don't necessarily need to go to a gym or lift weights. Instead, you can work out at home using resistance bands, household objects like bottles and cans, or your own body weight. Watching videos from reputable sources or working with a personal trainer can teach you what exercises to do and how to do them properly. Another good resource (if I do say so myself!) is my book *Fitter Faster*, which has step-by-step routines for all fitness levels, with an emphasis on slashing your workout time.

By building confidence, proper guidance can help overcome intimidation about exercise, including uncertainty over what to do and fears of getting hurt or looking silly. This apprehension, which I've experienced myself, can be a deterrent to exercise, especially among people who are heavy.

Another common barrier is a lack of time. To fit exercise into your day, make it a priority and schedule it just as you would a meeting or dinner with friends. Though you may have heard that early is ideal, the best time to exercise is actually whenever you can do it, whether that's morning, afternoon, or evening.

To boost your motivation, consider teaming up with a friend, which can make exercise more enjoyable and keep you more accountable because someone is expecting you. Many people find that fitness classes offer the same benefits.

Staying motivated also requires remembering why you're working out. As I said in chapter 3, viewing exercise mainly as a weight-control strategy often backfires. Instead, focus on how it improves your well-being, whether that means less stress, more energy, sounder sleep, or a greater sense of empowerment. By remaining mindful of such benefits, you can transform exercise over time from something you have to do into something you want to do, and thereby help ensure that you'll continue with it long term.

Sleep is another component of a healthy lifestyle that may affect your weight. A number of observational studies have linked insufficient sleep to obesity and weight gain. For example, in a study that followed more than 68,000 women for 16 years, researchers found that participants who routinely slept five hours a night were 32 percent more likely to gain at least 30 pounds than those who slept seven or eight hours. Women sleeping six hours also had a higher risk of weight gain.

These findings are supported by experimental research, including a study that assigned 200 subjects to sleep for only four hours a night in a lab for five consecutive nights. A control group slept in the lab for up to 10 hours every night. The sleep-restricted subjects put on an average of about 2 pounds, while the controls gained virtually no weight.

Pooling results from this trial and 10 others, researchers found that sleeping too little leads people to consume an extra 385 calories a day on average. Though scientists aren't sure why, there are several theories. One is that sleep deprivation affects the appetite-related hormones ghrelin and leptin, causing us to be hungrier. Some studies, but not all, support this idea. Sleep restriction may also affect our brains in other ways, dialing down activity in areas that control the impulse to eat, while activating reward centers that prompt us to seek out food. It's also possible that being awake more hours simply gives us more opportunity to eat. In addition, insufficient sleep has been shown to make the body less sensitive to insulin, which may spur fat storage.

Overall, research suggests that getting adequate sleep can be beneficial for not only your weight but also your overall health. Too little sleep is associated with a number of conditions, including diabetes, high blood pressure, heart disease, strokes, depression, and premature death. In addition, it impairs memory, attention, and concentration, which can lead to accidents.

Though people's sleep needs differ, most of us require seven to nine hours a night. Work and family obligations can make that a challenge, but a few simple strategies may help. For starters, put away your cell phone and other electronic devices an hour before bed. That way, you won't be tempted to stay up late texting, watching videos, or scrolling through Facebook. Also, try to go to sleep and wake up at the same times every day. Avoid alcohol and heavy meals right before bedtime, and keep your bedroom dark and quiet. If you have a condition like sleep apnea or depression that interferes with sleep, get treatment.

The third piece of a healthy lifestyle is stress management. When we're stressed, our adrenal glands pump out the hormone cortisol. If our stress is chronic, cortisol levels may remain high, contributing to weight gain in several possible ways. To begin with, elevated cortisol can promote the storage of abdominal fat, which as previously discussed is linked to health risks. A study involving more than 2,500 people aged 54 and up found that higher cortisol levels, as measured by hair analysis, were associated with larger waists, higher weights, and obesity. Though this doesn't prove cause and effect, we know that people with a condition called Cushing's syndrome, which involves an excess of cortisol, often experience weight gain, especially around the waist.

In addition, cortisol can affect weight by prompting us to eat more, with some people craving comfort foods like ice cream and pizza that are high in sugar and fat. In an American Psychological Association survey of nearly 2,000 adults, 38 percent reported overeating or succumbing to unhealthy foods in the past month because of stress. Women were especially likely to be affected.

Of course, not everyone responds to stress the same way. While some people eat more, others may eat less, and still others don't change their eating patterns. How you react may depend on certain personality traits as well as the nature of the stress. All of this, along with the fact that stress can be hard to measure, makes it tricky to study the relationship of stress with eating and weight. As a result, the evidence isn't ironclad. But it's strong enough to suggest that reducing stress may help with weight control, at least for some people.

Relaxation techniques such as yoga, meditation, and deep breathing can be effective for managing stress. Listening to music, playing with a pet, or spending time outdoors in nature may also help. Getting sufficient sleep is essential for controlling stress, and for many people, regular exercise is also key. (It certainly is for me.) If you're less stressed, you may be more likely to exercise and sleep better. In such a way, these three elements of a healthy lifestyle—exercise, sleep, and stress management—reinforce each other to benefit not only our physical and emotional health but also our weight.

Suanne's Journey

Growing up, Suanne wasn't overweight, but when her older sister went on a diet, so did Suanne. She recalls as a teen constantly being hungry due to restrictive diets and adopting an "all-or-nothing" mindset: She would either follow the diet to the letter or overindulge by, say, eating a tray of brownies. That was the beginning, she says, of her diet mentality, which would dominate her life for decades.

After struggling with weight gain throughout college, Suanne shed 50 pounds her senior year with the help of a commercial weight-loss program. But eventually, she started binge eating, and the weight returned. It was a pattern that continued for years. She would go on a restrictive diet and lose a lot of weight, then binge eat and regain it. And then diet again.

Tired of being trapped in this cycle, Suanne eventually gave up dieting. The bingeing stopped, but she felt overweight and out of shape, and had developed high blood pressure. This time, she adopted an eating plan she could stick with that didn't entail the restrictions of the diets she had previously followed. She lost about 30 pounds and lowered her blood pressure, which allowed her to cut back on the medication she was taking to control it. Though she experienced some setbacks during the COVID-19 pandemic, she managed to get back on track relatively quickly.

Today, Suanne focuses on filling up with vegetables and doesn't feel deprived. She exercises four or five times a week, either walking outdoors or working out at home with YouTube videos. Instead of seeing exercise as a way to burn off pounds, as she previously did, she's come to view it as a way to feel better.

Now in her 50s, Suanne has gained some key insights from her experiences: Restriction doesn't work for her. Any plan she follows has to be adaptable to her likes and dislikes, or it won't succeed. And weight control isn't just about what she eats; it's also about her mindset.

Though she's happy to have finally reached this place, she regrets all the years she spent dieting and obsessing over food. "I wish I knew then," she says, "what I know now."

Keep on Trackin'

Another proven strategy, self-monitoring, can involve keeping track of several things, including weight. As mentioned in the previous chapter, research shows that people who frequently weigh themselves are more likely to lose weight and keep it off than those who step on the scale only occasionally or never. A study of successful losers in the NWCR found that about 80 percent reported weighing themselves at least once a week, and 35 percent at least once a day. Frequent weighing is thought to help by allowing people to detect small gains and take action to reverse them before they become big gains. Weighing can also provide positive reinforcement, showing evidence of progress and motivating people to stick with dietary and lifestyle measures.

But as I also discussed, frequent weighing isn't for everyone. For some, it can cause psychological harm or contribute to an obsession with weight. Day-to-day weight fluctuations, which often stem from body water or hormonal changes, may be unduly discouraging (or encouraging) if they're not interpreted properly.

Whether regular weighing is helpful—and if so, the frequency that's optimal—are determinations that individuals have to make for themselves based on trial and error as well as their previous experiences with weight loss. In addition to (or instead of) weight, some people find it helpful to track metrics such as waist size, body fat, or clothing sizes.

Self-monitoring also includes recording what you eat. A number of apps aid in doing this, but they're not essential. If you prefer, you can enter the information in your computer or write it down in a notebook.

However you do it, keeping a food journal may improve both short-term and long-term weight loss, with people who are the most diligent about logging their information achieving the best results. That means recording every day, several times a day. Many of us can't recall what we ate this morning, much less last week. So food journals tend to be the most accurate—and therefore the most helpful—when you record what you eat and drink throughout the day rather than trying to do so hours or days later. One method is to note the information in your phone, which you can do quickly and inconspicuously, and then transfer it later.

Among the issues to track:

➲ **What and how much you ate or drank.** Be as specific as possible and include even small snacks, like a piece of candy. Some people find it helpful to take photos.

- ➲ **When you ate or drank.** What time was it? How close to waking up or going to bed?

- ➲ **Where you were.** At your kitchen table? At your desk? In a restaurant? At a party?

- ➲ **Whom you were with, if anyone.** Friends? Family? Colleagues?

- ➲ **What you were doing while eating or drinking.** Working? Watching TV? Driving? Visiting with others?

- ➲ **How you felt.** Were you stressed? Bored? Happy? Lonely? Tired? And how did you feel emotionally and physically after you ate or drank?

You may have noticed one item not listed here: calorie counts. That's because, as discussed in chapter 2, counting calories can be onerous, especially for home-cooked meals and foods served by friends or at social gatherings. Apps help, but only so much, and trying to deconstruct foods to figure out calorie counts can be time-consuming and frustrating.

A study that surveyed food journalers found recording calories to be high on the list of challenges. "It was difficult to estimate the amounts of each ingredient," said one respondent, "then find the calories (which weren't available for many of the foods I ate)." Some participants reported that this hassle negatively affected their food choices, with comments such as "The time it took . . . made eating fresh and healthy less appealing. Easier to scan a code on some processed stuff and be done with it."

If you want to track calories—or, for that matter, carbs, protein, and fat (a.k.a. macronutrients, or "macros")—that's fine as long as it doesn't undermine your efforts to keep a food journal or eat a healthful diet. The most important thing is to keep tabs on your eating patterns, which you can accomplish without crunching numbers.

Think of a journal as an awareness-raising tool. This can be helpful because we're not always fully aware of our eating habits. Our brains have a way of deceiving us, and journaling can provide a more objective record. For example, you might say—and honestly believe—"I hardly ever eat desserts" but learn through a journal that you grab sugary treats throughout the day at work. Or you might discover that, without realizing it at the time, you picked up fried food from the drive-through three times during an especially stressful week. Armed with a better understanding of what, when, and why you're eating, you can zero in on where you need to make changes. And you can see where you're improving or achieving your goals.

For a journal to be effective, you need to be honest when entering the information. Sometimes people shade the truth because they're ashamed of what they consumed or don't want to feel judged for "failing" in some way. But journals aren't and shouldn't be about shame, judgment, or failure. They're about empowering you with information that you can act on in the future. If your entries aren't accurate and complete, what you learn will, by definition, be inaccurate and incomplete, preventing you from reaping the full benefits of your journaling efforts.

As you get started, keeping a food journal may take more time, but eventually it should require only a few minutes a day. Be sure to allot time periodically to sit down and review the information. Some people find it helpful to continue journaling indefinitely, while others may need to do it for only a short time or during periods when they aren't seeing the results they want.

In addition to your eating habits, tracking your exercise, sleep, or stress levels, at least during certain periods, can also be useful. But not all forms of self-monitoring are necessary or helpful for everyone. By trying different types of tracking—and sticking with them long enough to assess their value—you can determine which are most beneficial for you.

Strategic Planning

It goes without saying that challenges are inevitable when it comes to weight control, so it's important to have plans in place to deal with some of the most common ones. Such plans, known in psychology as *implementation intentions*, include if-then statements: "If X happens, then I will do Y." The idea is that when faced with potential difficulties, we're ready with automatic responses that don't require decision-making or willpower. In a way, they're like auto technology that takes over the steering wheel to keep a drifting car in its lane. Research suggests that implementation intentions can keep us from veering off course and increase the likelihood of achieving our goals.

One obvious challenge is living in a society that tempts us with food seemingly everywhere we go, from pharmacies and filling stations to offices and airports. Resisting those M&M's constantly calling our name at the counter or Cheez-Its beckoning us from the vending machine can be tough, but having a plan may help. For some people, that might mean always keeping healthy snacks like fruit or carrot sticks with them that serve as readily available alternatives. Or perhaps they distract themselves by, say, texting a friend or checking e-mail when confronted with junk food in a checkout line. Whatever the strategies, the point is to be ready with predetermined responses.

Planning ahead can also help with the challenge of giant restaurant portions. We tend to eat whatever amount of food is in front of us, so relying on willpower to limit consumption is often ineffective. A go-to strategy might be to split a large entrée with a fellow diner or put part of it in a doggy bag at the *beginning* of the meal. Likewise, if you're attending a social gathering with lots of food, eating a filling snack beforehand and steering clear of the food table may help curtail the temptation to overindulge.

When it comes to eating at home, a lack of time may prompt you to regularly order pizza or pick up fast food instead of preparing a healthful meal. One solution might be to stock your freezer with nutritious meals (either packaged or made ahead of time) that are ready to eat in minutes. Or have ingredients handy that you can use to quickly throw together preset meals when you're in a pinch.

If the challenge is eating between meals, having healthful, effortless options like fruit or precut veggie sticks and hummus can be an effective strategy, as can keeping unhealthy snack foods like cookies and chips out of the house so you won't be tempted.

For those prone to emotional eating, using the "if/then" statement "If I feel the urge to eat, then I will rate my hunger" may be helpful. On a scale of 1 to 10, assess your hunger level. If you're truly hungry, eat a healthful snack. But if you're not and your desire to eat is driven more by stress, boredom, loneliness, or other feelings, the plan might be to go for a walk, listen to music, or call a friend instead.

In short, the more you can anticipate challenges and plan ahead for them, the less likely you'll wind up in a position to make food choices you'll regret. A food journal can be a useful tool for identifying these challenges and figuring out which strategies are most effective for you.

Even the best-laid plans, however, won't completely prevent setbacks. We all experience times when, for any number of reasons, we get derailed. Here, too, planning can make a difference. Research suggests that being armed with coping strategies can help prevent us from becoming discouraged and giving up when we have lapses.

In one study, researchers surveyed nearly 5,000 members of WW (formerly Weight Watchers) who had maintained weight loss of at least 20 pounds for more than three years. Their experiences were compared with those of a control group of people with obesity whose weights had remained the same. One of the key differences was that the successful losers were more likely to have psychological coping strategies such as "If I got off track, I encouraged myself by thinking positively" and "If I regained weight, I thought about my past successes and reminded myself that I could get back on track."

These folks didn't beat themselves up when they had setbacks. Instead, says the study's lead author, "they know there will be ups and downs, and they have a plan for coping with lapses that's empowering."

Expecting perfection is unrealistic and can lead to a self-defeating mindset—"I slipped, so I'm a failure"—that makes you less likely to persevere and achieve your goal. Instead, assume you'll fall off the horse along the way. When you do, being prepared with effective strategies can help you get back on and keep going.

Call in the Cavalry

Sometimes, despite our best efforts, self-help isn't sufficient, and we need to enlist the aid of professionals. One way is through what's known as *intensive behavioral therapy*, or IBT, which focuses on changing behaviors that contribute to obesity. Working with a health professional such as a therapist, physician, nurse practitioner, or registered dietitian, individuals seeking to lose weight receive guidance and support for issues like devising eating and exercise plans, setting goals, self-monitoring, identifying challenges, and developing strategies to deal with them. People can undergo IBT one-on-one or via group sessions, typically once a week at first, then once or twice a month. It can also be done online.

The US Preventive Services Task Force, which evaluates the evidence for various tests and treatments, looked at nearly 90 trials involving behavioral therapy and gave it a thumbs-up. The review found that after 12 to 18 months, people with obesity receiving behavioral counseling were nearly twice as likely to have shed 5 percent or more of their body weight compared with those in control groups. The behavioral therapy recipients also regained less weight and had a lower risk of developing diabetes. IBT may have similar benefits for people who are overweight but not obese.

Medicare and other insurance plans cover behavioral therapy for those with obesity if it's delivered through a primary care setting. You can also find elements of IBT in some commercial weight-loss programs. If you're interested in trying IBT, talk to your primary care provider.

Weight-loss (or bariatric) surgery is another effective option for certain people. To be eligible, someone typically needs to have a BMI over 40, or a BMI of at least 35 along with obesity-related conditions such as diabetes.

There are several types of bariatric procedures. The gold standard, known as *Roux-en-Y gastric bypass*, involves using the upper part of the stomach to create a small pouch about the size of an egg. The pouch is reconnected to the small intestine, bypassing the intestine's upper portion and therefore reducing the number of calories the gut absorbs. A less complicated and more common operation called *sleeve gastrectomy* reduces the stomach to the size of a banana. As with gastric bypass, this limits the amount of food someone can eat. Plus, sleeve gastrectomy removes an area of the stomach where most of the hunger hormone ghrelin is produced.

Research shows that bariatric surgery results in substantially greater weight loss than what's typically achieved with nonsurgical methods. For example, in a study that included more than 1,100 subjects with severe obesity who either did or did not undergo gastric bypass, the surgical group had lost an average of 35 percent of their initial weight after 2 years and 27 percent at 12 years. In contrast, the nonsurgical subjects' weights at 12 years were close to where they had started.

Surgery can produce dramatic improvements in health as well. In the aforementioned study, 75 percent of surgery subjects who initially had diabetes were free of the condition at two years, and half of them were still in remission at 12 years. What's more, those without diabetes who underwent surgery were far less likely to develop the disease than nonsurgery subjects. This and other research shows that surgery also improves high blood pressure, abnormal cholesterol, sleep apnea, and other conditions. And it's associated with reduced risks of cancer and premature death.

Though the safety of bariatric surgery has improved greatly in recent years, it nevertheless does have risks and possible side effects, including infection, blood clots, bowel obstruction, internal bleeding, leaks in the digestive tract, hernias, gallstones, vomiting, nausea, diarrhea, and acid reflux. In some cases, complications necessitate additional surgery.

Anyone considering surgery needs to carefully assess how these risks stack up against their weight-related health risks and the potential benefits of surgery. One factor that shouldn't enter the equation—but sometimes does—is the misguided notion that surgery is an easy way out. In fact, people undergoing surgery still need to make diet and lifestyle changes to achieve long-term success. Surgery simply provides a boost.

Weight loss is a battle against our biology, so we should welcome any effective ammunition that health professionals can arm us with—including surgery and behavioral therapy. The hope is that eventually medical science will be able to develop customized weight-control treatments, taking into account genetic, physiological, behavioral, social, and environmental factors to determine which approaches are most effective for which individuals. Research is under way on this strategy, known as *precision medicine*, but it's still in the early stages.

Weighing the Claims

For now, each of us has to determine for ourselves which approaches to weight loss are most effective. The principles described in this chapter are a good place to start. In addition, it's helpful to know how to make sense of the deluge of information about weight control and avoid falling for hype, half-truths, and myths. Here are eight tips to keep in mind.

➲ **1. Watch out for hyperbolic language.** If you encounter promises of rapid or guaranteed results, secrets, miracles, breakthroughs, effortless weight loss, or anything else that's too good to be true, assume that it is.

➲ **2. Ignore weight-loss advice from celebrities and self-appointed experts on social media.** Just because they're famous, have large followings, or sound persuasive doesn't mean they know what they're talking about and are qualified to give advice.

⊃ **3. Scrutinize the science.** When news reports, ads, or other sources refer to research, look for crucial details, including the type of research (e.g., in animals or human beings), how large the study was, how long it lasted, who was studied, and where it was published. If you're so inclined, look up the study on Google Scholar or Pubmed. gov. And even if the research is legitimate, don't base decisions on a single study.

⊃ **4. Don't be swayed by "before and after" photos.** Such images may be fake. The same goes for user testimonials. Even when these are real, they're often outliers and don't represent most people's experiences.

⊃ **5. Read the fine print.** Sometimes claims come with buried caveats such as "when combined with diet and exercise" or "these statements have not been evaluated by the Food and Drug Administration." Consider such disclaimers a red flag.

⊃ **6. Beware of experts who sell products.** Those who give advice and benefit financially from it by selling foods, supplements, or tests have a conflict of interest, which calls their credibility into question.

⊃ **7. Trust but verify.** Even if advice comes from someone with impressive-sounding degrees or academic affiliations, don't automatically take his or her word for it. Confirm the information with sources that objectively review the science, such as the Nutrition Source from the Harvard School of Public Health, *Nutrition Action Newsletter, U.S.*

News & World Report's annual "Best Diets" rankings, and Consumerlab.com.

➲ **8. Be suspicious of simple solutions.** Weight control is complex, involving a number of different factors. Anyone who claims to have a simple answer is denying reality, bending the truth, or both.

Heeding these suggestions can help prevent time-wasting, costly, and potentially dangerous detours on your weight-loss journey. Though the road is almost always winding and bumpy in places, with dead ends and loops that sometimes take you backward, here's hoping that what you've read in this book can serve as a GPS to keep you on the safest, most direct route to your destination. I wish you all the best on your trip.

ACKNOWLEDGMENTS

This project has been marinating in my mind for years. Without the help of a number of people, the idea would never have been served up as a book.

I'm enormously indebted to my friend and colleague Loren Goldfarb, who did a superb job (as he does in all his endeavors) as publisher, ably attending to every detail large and small, and assembling a first-rate team. That includes eagle-eyed editor Beth Bazar and talented designers Alex Head and Michael Rehder.

I'm also extremely grateful to the folks who were kind enough to share their inspiring journeys, and to Leigh Seaman, Mria Dangerfield, and Macie Goldfarb, who helped gather and/or write those stories.

A big thank-you as well to David Allison and Christopher Steele, both of whom generously lent their expertise, providing information and insights that were invaluable.

As always, my friend Lisa Lillien offered indispensable guidance and feedback, as did Erin Norcross, who served as a sounding board and patiently answered my many questions as I was writing the book.

Edward Felsenthal and my sister, Emily Weaver, made excellent suggestions that helped improve the manuscript. The same goes for my mom, Scottie, who carefully read every chapter and let me know what she did and didn't like. She's had a guiding hand in everything I've had published since age 9, when I penned a story for a children's magazine about a boy who encounters a monster on another planet. No words are adequate to thank her.

ENDNOTES

Introduction

2 *"Sing Sing prison inmates"*: Yager S. *The Hundred Year Diet: America's Voracious Appetite for Losing Weight.* New York: Rodale. 2010; 13.

3 *A groundbreaking paper:* Casazza K, Fontaine KR, Astrup A, et al. "Myths, Presumptions, and Facts about Obesity." *New England Journal of Medicine.* 2013; 368(5): 446–54.

3 *"nonsense and conjecture"*: telephone interview, Nov. 11, 2020.

3 *government surveys:* Han L, You D, Zeng F, et al. "Trends in Self-Perceived Weight Status, Weight Loss Attempts, and Weight Loss Strategies among Adults in the United States, 1999–2016." *JAMA Network Open.* 2019; 2(11): e1915219; Martin CB, Herrick KA, Sarafrazi N, et al. "Attempts to Lose Weight among Adults in the United States, 2013–2016." *NCHS Data Brief.* 2018; (313).

3 *Three-quarters report:* The ASMBS and NORC Survey on Obesity in America. American Society for Metabolic and Bariatric Surgery; NORC at the University of Chicago. 2016. https://www.norc.org/Research/Projects/Pages/the-asmbsnorc-obesity-poll.aspx

3 *worth more than $60 billion:* "The US Weight Loss & Diet Control Market." Researchandmarkets.com. 2021; March.

3-4 *42 percent of US adults now have obesity:* Hales CM, Carroll MD, Fryar CD, et al. "Prevalence of Obesity and Severe Obesity among Adults: United States, 2017–2018." *NCHS Data Brief.* 2020; (360).

4 *no state had an obesity rate over 20 percent:* Warren M, Beck S, Delgado D. "State of Obesity: Better Policies for a Healthier America." Trust for America's Health. 2020; Sept.

4 *obesity rate among children and adolescents:* Fryar CD, Carroll MD, Ogden CL. "Prevalence of Overweight, Obesity, and Severe Obesity among Adults Aged 20 and Over: United States, 1960–1962 through 2015–2016." NCHS Health E-Stats. 2018; Sept.

4 *70 percent of American adults: Health, United States, 2018.* National Center for Health Statistics. 2019. Table 21.

4 *Worldwide:* "Obesity and Overweight." World Health Organization. 2020. https://www.who.int/news-room/fact-sheets/detail/obesity-and-overweight

4 *dieters gain back more than half:* Anderson JW, Konz EC, Frederich RC, et al. "Long-Term Weight-Loss Maintenance: A Meta-Analysis of US Studies." *American Journal of Clinical Nutrition.* 2001; 74(5): 579–84.

4 *97 percent of people:* Kramer FM, Jeffery RW, Forster JL, et al. "Long-Term Follow-Up of Behavioral Treatment for Obesity: Patterns of Weight Regain among Men and Women." *International Journal of Obesity.* 1989; 13(2): 123–36.

5 *"might not have actually implemented":* Han, op cit.

9 *same types of exaggerations and omissions:* Woloshin S, Schwartz LM, Casella SL, et al. "Press Releases by Academic Medical Centers: Not So Academic?" *Annals of Internal Medicine.* 2009; 150(9): 613–8.

9 *studies sponsored by the food industry:* Sacks G, Riesenberg D, Mialon M, et al. "The Characteristics and Extent of Food Industry Involvement in Peer-Reviewed Research Articles from 10 Leading Nutrition-Related Journals in 2018." *PLOS One.* 2020; 15(12): e0243144.

10 *host of serious health problems:* "Health Risks of Overweight & Obesity." National Institute of Diabetes and Digestive and Kidney Diseases. https:// www.niddk.nih.gov/health-information/weight-management/adult-overweight-obesity/health-risks; Anstey KJ, Cherbuin N, Budge M, et al. "Body Mass Index in Midlife and Late-Life as a Risk Factor for Dementia: A Meta-Analysis of Prospective Studies." *Obesity Reviews.* 2011; May; 12(5): e426–37; Yu E, Ley SH, Manson JE, et al. "Weight History and All-Cause and Cause-Specific Mortality in Three Prospective Cohort Studies." *Annals of Internal Medicine.* 2017; 166(9): 613–20.

10 *flu and COVID-19:* Luzi L, Radaelli MG. "Influenza and Obesity: Its Odd Relationship and the Lessons for COVID-19 Pandemic." *Acta Diabetologica.* 2020; 57: 759–64; Pranata R, Lim MA, Yonas E, et al. "Body Mass Index and Outcome in Patients with COVID-19: A Dose–Response Meta-Analysis." *Diabetes & Metabolism.* 2021; 47(2): 101178.

10 *gaining as little as 10 pounds:* Zheng Y, Manson JE, Yuan C, et al. "Associations of Weight Gain from Early to Middle Adulthood with Major Health Outcomes Later in Life." *JAMA.* 2017; 318(3): 255–69.

10 *putting on 20 or more pounds:* Park SY, Wilkens LR, Maskarinec G, et al. "Weight Change in Older Adults and Mortality: The Multiethnic Cohort Study." *International Journal of Obesity.* 2018; 42(2): 205–12.

11 *75 percent of respondents:* The ASMBS and NORC Survey on Obesity in America. American Society for Metabolic and Bariatric Surgery; NORC at the University of Chicago. 2016. https://www.norc.org/Research/Projects/Pages/the-asmbsnorc-obesity-poll.aspx

11 New York Times *column:* Brody J. "Half of Us Face Obesity, Dire Projections Show." *New York Times.* 2020; Feb. 10.

11 *"We have set them up":* Prologo JD. "A Doctor's Open Apology to Those Fighting Overweight and Obesity." *The Conversation.* 2020; Sept. 8. https://theconversation.com/a-doctors-open-apology-to-those-fighting-overweight-and-obesity-145017

12 *associated with depression, anxiety . . .:* Pearl RL, Puhl RM. "Weight Bias Internalization and Health: A Systematic Review." *Obesity Reviews.* 2018; 19(8): 1141–63.

Chapter 1

18 *"The notion that there's one causal food":* Freedhoff Y. *The Diet Fix: Why Diets Fail and How to Make Yours Work.* New York: Harmony Books. 2014; 50.

19 *white paper reviewing the facts:* Pett KD, Kahn J, Willett WC, et al. "Ancel Keys and the Seven Countries Study: An Evidence-Based Response to Revisionist Histories." True Health Initiative. 2017.

19 *studies in animals:* West DB, York B. "Dietary Fat, Genetic Predisposition, and Obesity: Lessons from Animal Models." *American Journal of Clinical Nutrition.* 1998; 67(3): 505S–12S.

20 *Healthy People 2000:* US Office of Disease Prevention and Health Promotion. 1990.

21 *had "worked out very well":* Pennington AW. "A Reorientation on Obesity." *New England Journal of Medicine.* 1953; 248(23): 959–64.

22 *"Each time the diet has reappeared":* Schwartz H. *Never Satisfied: A Cultural History of Diets, Fantasies and Fat.* New York: Free Press. 1986; 8.

22 *"Would the gluten-free diet trend":* Fitzgerald, M. *Diet Cults: The Surprising Fallacy at the Core of Nutrition Fads and a Guide to Healthy Eating for the Rest of Us.* New York: Pegasus. 2014; 124.

22 *causes body fat to increase in mice:* Freire RH, Fernandes LR, Silva RB, et al. "Wheat Gluten Intake Increases Weight Gain and Adiposity Associated with Reduced Thermogenesis and Energy Expenditure in an Animal Model of Obesity." *International Journal of Obesity.* 2016; 40(3): 479–86.

23 *today's wheat is more fattening:* Brouns FJ, van Buul VJ, Shewry PR. "Does Wheat Make Us Fat and Sick?" *Journal of Cereal Science.* 2013; 58(2): 209–15.

23 *research by Ludwig:* Ebbeling CB, Feldman HA, Klein GL, et al. "Effects of a Low Carbohydrate Diet on Energy Expenditure during Weight Loss Maintenance: Randomized Trial." *BMJ.* 2018; 363.

23 *metabolic rates didn't increase as predicted:* Hall KD. "A Review of the Carbohydrate-Insulin Model of Obesity." *European Journal of Clinical Nutrition.* 2017; 71(3): 323–6.

23-4 *pooled results from more than 20 population studies:* Sartorius K, Sartorius B, Madiba TE, et al. "Does High-Carbohydrate Intake Lead to Increased Risk of Obesity? A Systematic Review and Meta-Analysis." *BMJ Open.* 2018; 8(2): e018449.

24 *study published in the* New England Journal of Medicine*:* Sacks FM, Bray GA, Carey VJ, et al. "Comparison of Weight-Loss Diets with Different Compositions of Fat, Protein, and Carbohydrates." *New England Journal of Medicine.* 2009; 360(9): 859–73.

24 *An* Annals of Internal Medicine *study:* Foster GD, Wyatt HR, Hill JO, et al. "Weight and Metabolic Outcomes after 2 Years on a Low-Carbohydrate versus Low-Fat Diet: A Randomized Trial." *Annals of Internal Medicine.* 2010; 153(3): 147–57.

25 *study known as DIETFITS:* Gardner CD, Trepanowski JF, Del Gobbo LC, et al. "Effect of Low-Fat vs Low-Carbohydrate Diet on 12-Month Weight Loss in Overweight Adults and the Association with Genotype Pattern or Insulin Secretion: The DIETFITS Randomized Clinical Trial." *JAMA.* 2018; 319(7): 667–79.

25 *low-carb diets may be more effective:* Mansoor N, Vinknes KJ, Veierød MB, et al. "Effects of Low-Carbohydrate Diets v. Low-Fat Diets on Body Weight and Cardiovascular Risk Factors: A Meta-Analysis of Randomised Controlled Trials." *British Journal of Nutrition.* 2016; 115(3): 466–79; Hession M, Rolland C, Kulkarni U, et al. "Systematic Review of Randomized Controlled Trials of Low-Carbohydrate vs. Low-Fat/Low-Calorie Diets in the Management of Obesity and Its Comorbidities." *Obesity Reviews.* 2009; 10(1): 36–50.

25 *insulin status may play a role:* Ebbeling CB, Leidig MM, Feldman HA, et al. "Effects of a Low–Glycemic Load vs Low-Fat Diet in Obese Young Adults: A Randomized Trial." *JAMA.* 2007; 297(19): 2092–102; Cornier MA, Donahoo WT, Pereira R, et al. "Insulin Sensitivity Determines the Effectiveness of Dietary Macronutrient Composition on Weight Loss in Obese Women." *Obesity Research.* 2005; 13(4): 703–9.

26 *trials comparing Ornish to Atkins:* Gardner CD, Kiazand A, Alhassan S, et al. "Comparison of the Atkins, Zone, Ornish, and LEARN Diets for Change in Weight and Related Risk Factors among Overweight Premenopausal Women: The A to Z Weight Loss Study: A Randomized Trial." *JAMA.* 2007; 297(9): 969–77; Dansinger ML, Gleason JA, Griffith JL, et al. "Comparison of the Atkins, Ornish, Weight Watchers, and Zone Diets for Weight Loss and Heart Disease Risk Reduction: A Randomized Trial." *JAMA.* 2005; 293(1): 43–53.

26 *study that pooled results from 13 trials:* Bueno NB, de Melo IS, de Oliveira SL, et al. "Very-Low-Carbohydrate Ketogenic Diet v. Low-Fat Diet for Long-Term Weight Loss: A Meta-Analysis of Randomised Controlled Trials." *British Journal of Nutrition.* 2013; 110(7): 1178–87.

27 *replacing carbs with lots of saturated fat:* Kirkpatrick CF, Bolick JP, Kris-Etherton PM, et al. "Review of Current Evidence and Clinical Recommendations on the Effects of Low-Carbohydrate and Very-Low-Carbohydrate (Including Ketogenic) Diets for the Management of Body Weight and Other Cardiometabolic Risk Factors: A Scientific Statement from the National Lipid Association Nutrition and Lifestyle Task Force." *Journal of Clinical Lipidology.* 2019; 13(5): 689–711.

29 *failed to show that low-GI or -GL diets are superior:* Vega-López S, Venn BJ, Slavin JL. "Relevance of the Glycemic Index and Glycemic Load for Body Weight, Diabetes, and Cardiovascular Disease." *Nutrients.* 2018; 10(10): 1361.

29-30 *video of the talk:* "Sugar: The Bitter Truth." https://www.youtube.com/watch?v=dBnniua6-oM

30 *"the primary . . . villain":* Lustig RH. *Fat Chance: Beating the Odds against Sugar, Processed Food, Obesity, and Disease.* New York: Avery. 2012; 21.

30 *studies of rodents:* Lê KA, Tappy L. "Metabolic Effects of Fructose." *Current Opinion in Clinical Nutrition & Metabolic Care.* 2006; 9(4): 469–75.

30-1 *study commissioned by the World Health Organization:* Te Morenga L, Mallard S, Mann J. "Dietary Sugars and Body Weight: Systematic Review and Meta-Analyses of Randomised Controlled Trials and Cohort Studies." *BMJ.* 2013; 346: e7492.

31 *extra pounds are due to extra calories:* van Buul VJ, Tappy L, Brouns FJ. "Misconceptions about Fructose-Containing Sugars and Their Role in the Obesity Epidemic." *Nutrition Research Reviews.* 2014; 27(1): 119–30.

31 *sugar intake among adults:* Marriott BP, Hunt KJ, Malek AM, et al. "Trends in Intake of Energy and Total Sugar from Sugar-Sweetened Beverages in the United States among Children and Adults, NHANES 2003–2016." *Nutrients.* 2019; 11(9): 2004.

31 *adult obesity rates:* Hales CM, Carroll MD, Fryar CD, et al. "Prevalence of Obesity among Adults and Youth: United States, 2015–2016." *NCHS Data Brief.* 2017; (288).

31 *no solid evidence that HFCS is any worse for us than sugar:* Moeller SM, Fryhofer SA, Osbahr III AJ, et al. "The Effects of High Fructose Syrup." *Journal of the American College of Nutrition.* 2009; 28(6): 619–26.

32 *limited evidence that these foods promote weight loss:* Borges MC, Louzada ML, de Sá TH, et al. "Artificially Sweetened Beverages and the Response to the Global Obesity Crisis." *PLOS Medicine.* 2017; 14(1): e1002195.

32 *research has even linked them to weight gain:* Azad MB, Abou-Setta AM, Chauhan BF, et al. "Nonnutritive Sweeteners and Cardiometabolic Health: A Systematic Review and Meta-Analysis of Randomized Controlled Trials and Prospective Cohort Studies." *CMAJ.* 2017; 189(28): E929–39.

32 *fruit does not contribute to weight gain:* Hebden L, O'Leary F, Rangan A, et al. "Fruit Consumption and Adiposity Status in Adults: A Systematic Review of Current Evidence." *Critical Reviews in Food Science and Nutrition.* 2017; 57(12): 2526–40.

32 *three large studies:* Bertoia ML, Mukamal KJ, Cahill LE, et al. "Changes in Intake of Fruits and Vegetables and Weight Change in United States Men and Women Followed for Up to 24 Years: Analysis from Three Prospective Cohort Studies." *PLOS Medicine.* 2015; 12(9).

32 *Research has linked it to weight gain:* Hebden, op cit.

33 *Groups with higher consumption of SSBs:* Rosinger A, Herrick KA, Gahche JJ, et al. "Sugar-Sweetened Beverage Consumption among U.S. Adults, 2011–2014." *NCHS Data Brief.* 2017; (270).

33 *video in which a man scarfed down globs of fat:* https://www.youtube.com/watch?v=-F4t8zL6F0c

33 *study examining 17 large reviews:* Bes-Rastrollo M, Schulze MB, Ruiz-Canela M, et al. "Financial Conflicts of Interest and Reporting Bias Regarding the Association between Sugar-Sweetened Beverages and Weight Gain: A Systematic Review of Systematic Reviews." *PLOS Medicine.* 2013; 10(12).

33-4 *team of Harvard researchers:* Malik VS, Pan A, Willett WC, et al. "Sugar-Sweetened Beverages and Weight Gain in Children and Adults: A Systematic Review and Meta-Analysis." *American Journal of Clinical Nutrition.* 2013; 98(4): 1084–102.

34 *consumption of SSBs has decreased:* Marriott, op cit.

34 *Rates continued their march upward:* Hales, op cit.

34 *taxes can decrease purchases of SSBs:* Bes-Rastrollo M, Sayon-Orea C, Ruiz-Canela M, et al. "Impact of Sugars and Sugar Taxation on Body Weight Control: A Comprehensive Literature Review." *Obesity.* 2016; 24(7): 1410–26.

36 *light to moderate consumption of beer:* Traversy G, Chaput JP. "Alcohol Consumption and Obesity: An Update." *Current Obesity Reports.* 2015; 4(1): 122–30.

36 *women who drink moderately:* Wang L, Lee IM, Manson JE, et al. "Alcohol Consumption, Weight Gain, and Risk of Becoming Overweight in Middle-Aged and Older Women." *Archives of Internal Medicine.* 2010; 170(5): 453–61.

36 *ONAAT fallacy:* Katz, D. "Why Holistic Nutrition Is the Best Approach." *HuffPost.* 2011; Apr. 1 https://www.huffpost.com/entry/holistic-nutrition_b_842627

37 *eating pattern is effective:* Laster J, Frame LA. "Beyond the Calories—Is the Problem in the Processing?" *Current Treatment Options in Gastroenterology.* 2019; Dec. 1; 17(4):577–86; Hall KD, Ayuketah A, Brychta R, et al. "Ultra-Processed Diets Cause Excess Calorie Intake and Weight Gain: An Inpatient Randomized Controlled Trial of Ad Libitum Food Intake." *Cell Metabolism.* 2019; 30(1): 67–77.

Chapter 2

42 *National Institutes of Health (NIH) website:* www.nhlbi.nih.gov/
health-topics/overweight-and-obesity

42 *World Health Organization:* www.who.int/en/news-room/fact-sheets/
detail/obesity-and-overweight

42 *Nutrition.gov site:* www.nutrition.gov/topics/healthy-weight/
strategies-success/interested-losing-weight

44 *"first modern nutrition scientist":* Nestle M, Nesheim M. *Why Calories
Count: From Science to Politics.* University of California Press. 2012; 32. Nestle
and Nesheim's book, which is dedicated to the memory of Atwater, provides
an excellent overview of his groundbreaking work.

45 *study of more than 200 foods:* Urban LE, McCrory MA, Dallal GE, et al.
"Accuracy of Stated Energy Contents of Restaurant Foods." *JAMA.* 2011;
306(3): 287–93.

45 *actual count, according to research, is 129:* Novotny JA, Gebauer SK,
Baer DJ. "Discrepancy between the Atwater Factor Predicted and Empirically
Measured Energy Values of Almonds in Human Diets." *American Journal of
Clinical Nutrition.* 2012; 96(2): 296–301.

45 *other nuts such as walnuts and cashews:* Baer DJ, Gebauer SK, Novotny
JA. "Walnuts Consumed by Healthy Adults Provide Less Available Energy
than Predicted by the Atwater Factors." *Journal of Nutrition.* 2016; 146(1):
9–13; Baer DJ, Novotny JA. "Metabolizable Energy from Cashew Nuts Is Less
Than That Predicted by Atwater Factors." *Nutrients.* 2018; 11(1): 33.

45 *mice ate meat and starchy foods:* Carmody RN, Weintraub GS, Wrangham
RW. "Energetic Consequences of Thermal and Nonthermal Food Processing."
Proceedings of the National Academy of Sciences USA. 2011; 108(48):
19199–203.

46 *foods such as celery:* Clegg ME, Cooper C. "Exploring the Myth: Does
Eating Celery Result in a Negative Energy Balance?" *Proceedings of the
Nutrition Society.* 2012; 71 (OCE3).

47 *number is likely too small:* Brown CM, Dulloo AG, Montani JP. "Water-
Induced Thermogenesis Reconsidered: The Effects of Osmolality and Water
Temperature on Energy Expenditure after Drinking." *Journal of Clinical
Endocrinology & Metabolism.* 2006; 91(9): 3598–602.

47 *survey of 2,200 adults:* National Tracking Poll #180615. Morning Consult.
2018.

47 *researchers asked 115 mall shoppers:* Lee WC, Shimizu M, Kniffin KM,
et al. "You Taste What You See: Do Organic Labels Bias Taste Perceptions?"
Food Quality and Preference. 2013; 29(1): 33–9.

47 *subjects were shown either a cheeseburger:* Chernev A, Gal D. "Categorization Effects in Value Judgments: Averaging Bias in Evaluating Combinations of Vices and Virtues." *Journal of Marketing Research.* 2010; 47(4): 738–47.

48 *survey of 1,000 people:* International Food Information Council Foundation. *Food & Health Survey: Consumer Attitudes toward Food Safety, Nutrition & Health.* 2012.

48 *Wearable devices:* Murakami H, Kawakami R, Nakae S, et al. "Accuracy of Wearable Devices for Estimating Total Energy Expenditure: Comparison with Metabolic Chamber and Doubly Labeled Water Method." *JAMA Internal Medicine.* 2016; 176(5): 702–3.

49 *"because it is too difficult to do precisely":* Nestle, op cit. 219.

50 *research shows that the hormone stays elevated:* Sumithran P, Prendergast LA, Delbridge E, et al. "Long-Term Persistence of Hormonal Adaptations to Weight Loss." *New England Journal of Medicine.* 2011; 365(17): 1597–604.

50 *other estimates:* Hall KD, Heymsfield SB, Kemnitz JW, et al. "Energy Balance and Its Components: Implications for Body Weight Regulation." *American Journal of Clinical Nutrition.* 2012; 95(4): 989–94.

51 *researchers locked up 12 pairs:* Bouchard C, Tremblay A, Després JP, et al. "The Response to Long-Term Overfeeding in Identical Twins." *New England Journal of Medicine.* 1990; 322(21): 1477–82.

51 *study of 14 pairs of obese female twins:* Hainer V, Stunkard AJ, Kunešová M, et al. "Intrapair Resemblance in Very Low Calorie Diet-Induced Weight Loss in Female Obese Identical Twins." *International Journal of Obesity.* 2000; 24(8): 1051–7.

51 *Further evidence comes from population studies:* Stryjecki C, Alyass A, Meyre D. "Ethnic and Population Differences in the Genetic Predisposition to Human Obesity." *Obesity Reviews.* 2018; 19(1): 62–80.

52 *gene-mapping studies:* Ibid.

52 *Pima Indians:* Schulz LO, Chaudhari LS. "High-Risk Populations: The Pimas of Arizona and Mexico." *Current Obesity Reports.* 2015; 4(1): 92–8.

53 *To show how gut microbes contribute to weight gain:* Turnbaugh PJ, Ley RE, Mahowald MA, et al. "An Obesity-Associated Gut Microbiome with Increased Capacity for Energy Harvest." *Nature.* 2006; 444(7122): 1027–31.

53 *In another experiment:* Ridaura VK, Faith JJ, Rey FE, et al. "Gut Microbiota from Twins Discordant for Obesity Modulate Metabolism in Mice." *Science.* 2013; 341(6150): 1241214.

53 *There's anecdotal evidence:* Alang N, Kelly CR. "Weight Gain after Fecal Microbiota Transplantation." *Open Forum Infectious Diseases.* 2015; 2(1).

54 *birth control pills:* Gallo MF, Lopez LM, Grimes DA, et al. "Combination Contraceptives: Effects on Weight." *Cochrane Database of Systematic Reviews.* 2014; 1.

54 *linked antibiotic use to higher weights in children:* Schwartz BS, Pollak J, Bailey-Davis L, et al. "Antibiotic Use and Childhood Body Mass Index Trajectory." *International Journal of Obesity.* 2016; 40(4): 615–21.

54 *less evidence about the impact on adults:* Leong KS, Derraik JG, Hofman PL, et al. "Antibiotics, Gut Microbiome and Obesity." *Clinical Endocrinology.* 2018; 88(2): 185–200.

55 *research has failed to show:* Borges MC, Louzada ML, de Sá TH, et al. "Artificially Sweetened Beverages and the Response to the Global Obesity Crisis." *PLOS Medicine.* 2017; 14(1): e1002195; Azad MB, Abou-Setta AM, Chauhan BF, et al. "Nonnutritive Sweeteners and Cardiometabolic Health: A Systematic Review and Meta-Analysis of Randomized Controlled Trials and Prospective Cohort Studies." *CMAJ.* 2017; 189(28): E929–39.

55 *only certain artificial sweeteners:* Ruiz-Ojeda FJ, Plaza-Díaz J, Sáez-Lara MJ, et al. "Effects of Sweeteners on the Gut Microbiota: A Review of Experimental Studies and Clinical Trials." *Advances in Nutrition.* 2019; 10(suppl 1): S31–48.

56 *Research has associated it with a host of health problems:* Gardener H, Elkind MS. "Artificial Sweeteners, Real Risks." *Stroke.* 2019; 50(3): 549–51.

56 *Pooling results from 14 relatively rigorous studies:* Cantu-Jungles T, McCormack L, Slaven J, et al. "A Meta-Analysis to Determine the Impact of Restaurant Menu Labeling on Calories and Nutrients (Ordered or Consumed) in US Adults." *Nutrients.* 2017; 9(10): 1088.

56 *people with higher obesity rates:* Green JE, Brown AG, Ohri-Vachaspati P. "Sociodemographic Disparities among Fast-Food Restaurant Customers Who Notice and Use Calorie Menu Labels." *Journal of the Academy of Nutrition and Dietetics.* 2015; 115(7): 1093–101.

56 *order foods with more calories:* Downs JS, Wisdom J, Wansink B, et al. "Supplementing Menu Labeling with Calorie Recommendations to Test for Facilitation Effects." *American Journal of Public Health.* 2013; 103(9):1604–9.

57 *study of 1,800 young men and women:* Larson N, Haynos AF, Roberto CA, et al. "Calorie Labels on the Restaurant Menu: Is the Use of Weight-Control Behaviors Related to Ordering Decisions?" *Journal of the Academy of Nutrition and Dietetics.* 2018; 118(3): 399–408.

Chapter 3

63 *analysis of 66 episodes:* Klos LA, Greenleaf C, Paly N, et al. "Losing Weight on Reality TV: A Content Analysis of the Weight Loss Behaviors and Practices Portrayed on *The Biggest Loser.*" *Journal of Health Communication.* 2015; 20(6): 639–46.

64 *US government survey:* Martin CB, Herrick KA, Sarafrazi N, et al. "Attempts to Lose Weight among Adults in the United States, 2013–2016." *NCHS Data Brief.* 2018; (313).

65 *popular women's magazines:* "Stretch and Grow Slim" (*Ladies' Home Journal,* April 1928); "Ten Minutes a Day Keep the Bulges Away" (*Ladies' Home Journal,* July 1946); "Six Easy Exercises for the Bosom" (*Good Housekeeping,* May 1940). These and many other examples are cited in Shaulis DE. "Exercising Authority: A Critical History of Exercise Messages in Popular Magazines, 1925–1968." UNLV Dissertation. 1997.

66 *"The Best Diet Is Exercise":* Mayer J. "The Best Diet Is Exercise." *New York Times.* 1965; April 25.

68 *typically produces little or no weight loss:* Swift DL, McGee JE, Earnest CP, et al. "The Effects of Exercise and Physical Activity on Weight Loss and Maintenance." *Progress in Cardiovascular Diseases.* 2018; 61(2): 206–13.

68 *Pooling data from six trials:* Johns DJ, Hartmann-Boyce J, Jebb SA, et al. "Diet or Exercise Interventions vs Combined Behavioral Weight Management Programs: A Systematic Review and Meta-Analysis of Direct Comparisons." *Journal of the Academy of Nutrition and Dietetics.* 2014; 114(10): 1557–68.

68 *difference was less than 3 pounds:* Wu T, Gao X, Chen M, et al. "Long-Term Effectiveness of Diet-Plus-Exercise Interventions vs. Diet-Only Interventions for Weight Loss: A Meta-Analysis." *Obesity Reviews.* 2009; 10(3): 313–23.

68 *studies where exercise has produced meaningful weight loss:* Swift, op cit.

69 *one small study:* Knab AM, Shanely RA, Corbin KD, et al. "A 45-Minute Vigorous Exercise Bout Increases Metabolic Rate for 14 Hours." *Medicine & Science in Sports & Exercise.* 2011; 43(9): 1643–8.

69 *High-intensity interval training:* Moniz SC, Islam H, Hazell TJ. "Mechanistic and Methodological Perspectives on the Impact of Intense Interval Training on Post-Exercise Metabolism." *Scandinavian Journal of Medicine & Science In Sports.* 2020; 30(4): 638–51.

70 *study in which overweight subjects did supervised high-intensity exercise:* King NA, Hopkins M, Caudwell P, et al. "Individual Variability Following 12 Weeks of Supervised Exercise: Identification and Characterization of Compensation for Exercise-Induced Weight Loss." *International Journal of Obesity.* 2008; 32(1): 177–84.

71 *greater hunger and more cravings for sweets:* Martin CK, Johnson WD, Myers CA, et al. "Effect of Different Doses of Supervised Exercise on Food Intake, Metabolism, and Non-Exercise Physical Activity: The E-MECHANIC Randomized Controlled Trial." *American Journal of Clinical Nutrition.* 2019; 110(3): 583–92.

71 *estimated how many calories they had burned:* Willbond SM, Laviolette MA, Duval K, et al. "Normal Weight Men and Women Overestimate Exercise Energy Expenditure." *Journal of Sports Medicine and Physical Fitness.* 2010; 50(4): 377–84.

72 *show reductions in NEAT:* Manthou E, Gill JM, Wright A, et al. "Behavioral Compensatory Adjustments to Exercise Training in Overweight Women." *Medicine & Science in Sports & Exercise.* 2010; 42(6): 1121–8.

72 *study of overweight and obese women:* Hopkins M, Gibbons C, Caudwell P, et al. "The Adaptive Metabolic Response to Exercise-Induced Weight Loss Influences Both Energy Expenditure and Energy Intake." *European Journal of Clinical Nutrition.* 2014; 68(5): 581–6.

72-3 *total energy expenditure may plateau:* Pontzer H, Durazo-Arvizu R, Dugas LR, et al. "Constrained Total Energy Expenditure and Metabolic Adaptation to Physical Activity in Adult Humans." *Current Biology.* 2016; 26(3): 410–7.

73 *half of this variation is due to heredity:* Bouchard C, An P, Rice T, et al. "Familial Aggregation of VO_2 Max Response to Exercise Training: Results from the HERITAGE Family Study." *Journal of Applied Physiology.* 1999; 87(3): 1003–8.

74 *study of seven devices:* Shcherbina A, Mattsson CM, Waggott D, et al. "Accuracy in Wrist-Worn, Sensor-Based Measurements of Heart Rate and Energy Expenditure in a Diverse Cohort." *Journal of Personalized Medicine.* 2017; 7(2): 3.

74 *National Weight Control Registry:* Catenacci VA, Ogden LG, Stuht J, et al. "Physical Activity Patterns in the National Weight Control Registry." *Obesity.* 2008; 16(1): 153–61.

74 *study involving overweight women:* Jakicic JM, Marcus BH, Lang W, et al. "Effect of Exercise on 24-Month Weight Loss Maintenance in Overweight Women." *Archives of Internal Medicine.* 2008; 168(14): 1550–9.

74 *research involving 14 contestants on* The Biggest Loser: Kerns JC, Guo J, Fothergill E, et al. "Increased Physical Activity Associated with Less Weight Regain Six Years after 'The Biggest Loser' Competition." *Obesity.* 2017; 25(11): 1838–43.

75 *study that followed participants for 20 years:* Hankinson AL, Daviglus ML, Bouchard C, et al. "Maintaining a High Physical Activity Level over 20 Years and Weight Gain." *JAMA.* 2010: 304(23): 2603–10.

75 *study that gathered data on 19,000 Norwegians:* Moholdt T, Wisløff U, Lydersen S, et al. "Current Physical Activity Guidelines for Health Are Insufficient to Mitigate Long-Term Weight Gain: More Data in the Fitness versus Fatness Debate (The HUNT Study, Norway)." *British Journal of Sports Medicine.* 2014; 48(20): 1489–96.

75 *levels of at least 150 minutes a week:* Jakicic JM, Powell KE, Campbell WW, et al. "Physical Activity and the Prevention of Weight Gain in Adults: A Systematic Review." *Medicine & Science in Sports & Exercise.* 2019; 51(6): 1262–9; Swift, op cit.

76 *aerobic activities generally have a greater effect on weight:* Swift, op cit.

76 *can decrease body fat:* Drenowatz C, Hand GA, Sagner M, et al. "The Prospective Association between Different Types of Exercise and Body Composition." *Medicine & Science in Sports & Exercise.* 2015; 47(12): 2535–41.

77 *Combining data from more than 100 studies:* Verheggen RJ, Maessen MF, Green DJ, et al. "A Systematic Review and Meta-Analysis on the Effects of Exercise Training versus Hypocaloric Diet: Distinct Effects on Body Weight and Visceral Adipose Tissue." *Obesity Reviews.* 2016; 17(8): 664–90.

77 *Higher amounts of visceral fat:* Piché ME, Poirier P, Lemieux I, et al. "Overview of Epidemiology and Contribution of Obesity and Body Fat Distribution to Cardiovascular Disease: An Update." *Progress in Cardiovascular Diseases.* 2018; 61(2): 103–13.

77 *pooling data from 10 studies:* Barry VW, Baruth M, Beets MW, et al. "Fitness vs. Fatness on All-Cause Mortality: A Meta-Analysis." *Progress in Cardiovascular Diseases.* 2014; 56(4): 382–90.

77 *live longer than lean couch potatoes:* Lee CD, Blair SN, Jackson AS. "Cardiorespiratory Fitness, Body Composition, and All-Cause and Cardiovascular Disease Mortality in Men." *American Journal of Clinical Nutrition.* 1999; 69(3): 373–80.

78 *odds of developing risk factors:* Lee DC, Sui X, Church TS, et al. "Changes in Fitness and Fatness on the Development of Cardiovascular Disease Risk Factors: Hypertension, Metabolic Syndrome, and Hypercholesterolemia." *Journal of the American College of Cardiology.* 2012; 59(7): 665–72.

80 *this response was typical:* Guess N. "A Qualitative Investigation of Attitudes towards Aerobic and Resistance Exercise amongst Overweight and Obese Individuals." *BMC Research Notes.* 2012; 5: 191.

80 *write down their thoughts about physical activity:* Segar M, Spruijt-Metz D, Nolen-Hoeksema S. "Go Figure? Body-Shape Motives Are Associated with Decreased Physical Activity Participation among Midlife Women." *Sex Roles.* 2006; 54(3–4): 175–87.

Chapter 4

85 *"you'll literally burn away your fat":* https://www.doctoroz.com/article/swimsuit-slimdown-plan

86 *"acidic nature of ACV helps stimulate":* Bragg P, Bragg PC. *Apple Cider Vinegar: Miracle Health System.* Bragg Health Sciences. 2008; 20.

86 *genes involved in the formation and breakdown of fat:* Petsiou EI, Mitrou PI, Raptis SA, et al. "Effect and Mechanisms of Action of Vinegar on Glucose Metabolism, Lipid Profile, and Body Weight." *Nutrition Reviews.* 2014; 72(10): 651–61.

86 *most frequently cited study:* Kondo T, Kishi M, Fushimi T, et al. "Vinegar Intake Reduces Body Weight, Body Fat Mass, and Serum Triglyceride Levels in Obese Japanese Subjects." *Bioscience, Biotechnology, and Biochemistry.* 2009; 73(8): 1837–43.

86 *may reduce spikes in blood sugar:* Shishehbor F, Mansoori A, Shirani F. "Vinegar Consumption Can Attenuate Postprandial Glucose and Insulin Responses; A Systematic Review and Meta-Analysis of Clinical Trials." *Diabetes Research and Clinical Practice.* 2017; 127: 1–9.

86 *may decrease appetite:* Darzi J, Frost GS, Montaser R, et al. "Influence of the Tolerability of Vinegar As an Oral Source of Short-Chain Fatty Acids on Appetite Control and Food Intake." *International Journal of Obesity.* 2014; 38(5): 675–81.

87 *concentration of acetic acid in ACV pills:* https://www.consumerlab.com/apple-cider-vinegar/

87 *resulted in greater weight loss:* Parretti HM, Aveyard P, Blannin A, et al. "Efficacy of Water Preloading before Main Meals As a Strategy for Weight Loss in Primary Care Patients with Obesity: RCT." *Obesity.* 2015; 23(9): 1785–91; Dennis EA, Dengo AL, Comber DL, et al. "Water Consumption Increases Weight Loss During a Hypocaloric Diet Intervention in Middle-Aged and Older Adults." *Obesity.* 2010; 18(2): 300–7.

87 *younger people:* Corney RA, Sunderland C, James LJ. "Immediate Pre-Meal Water Ingestion Decreases Voluntary Food Intake in Lean Young Males." *European Journal of Nutrition.* 2016; 55(2): 815–9.

88 *"Eat more of coconut oil":* Mercola J. "Eat More of Coconut Oil and You Might Slim Your Waist Size in One Week." Mercola.com. 2011; Dec. 29. https://articles.mercola.com/sites/articles/archive/2011/12/29/coconut-oil-slim-your-waist-size-in-one-week.aspx

88 *MCTs have been shown to increase fullness and rev up metabolism:* Clegg ME. "They Say Coconut Oil Can Aid Weight Loss, but Can It Really?" *European Journal of Clinical Nutrition.* 2017; 71(10): 1139–43.

88 *trials comparing MCTs with LCTs:* Mumme K, Stonehouse W. "Effects of Medium-Chain Triglycerides on Weight Loss and Body Composition: A Meta-Analysis of Randomized Controlled Trials." *Journal of the Academy of Nutrition and Dietetics.* 2015; 115(2): 249–63.

89 *One of the few published studies:* Assunçao ML, Ferreira HS, dos Santos AF, et al. "Effects of Dietary Coconut Oil on the Biochemical and Anthropometric Profiles of Women Presenting Abdominal Obesity." *Lipids.* 2009; 44(7): 593–601.

89 *Other small, short-term studies:* For example, see Vogel CÉ, Crovesy L, Rosado EL, et al. "Effect of Coconut Oil on Weight Loss and Metabolic Parameters in Men with Obesity: A Randomized Controlled Clinical Trial." *Food & Function.* 2020; 11(7): 6588–94.

89 *"unrealistic and unsupported by scientific evidence":* Lima RD, Block JM. "Coconut Oil: What Do We Really Know about It So Far?" *Food Quality and Safety.* 2019; 3(2): 61–72.

89 *saturated fat in coconut oil raises LDL:* Neelakantan N, Seah JY, van Dam RM. "The Effect of Coconut Oil Consumption on Cardiovascular Risk Factors: A Systematic Review and Meta-Analysis of Clinical Trials." *Circulation.* 2020; 141(10): 803–14.

90 *4 cups a day may modestly reduce body fat:* Alperet DJ, Rebello SA, Khoo EY, et al. "The Effect of Coffee Consumption on Insulin Sensitivity and Other Biological Risk Factors for Type 2 Diabetes: A Randomized Placebo-Controlled Trial." *American Journal of Clinical Nutrition.* 2020; 111(2): 448–58.

90 *"Avocados May Be the Key to Weight Loss, Study Says":* Martinez P. "Avocados May Be the Key to Weight Loss, Study Says." Foxnews. com. 2019; May 21. https://www.foxnews.com/food-drink/ avocados-may-key-weight-loss-study

90 *researchers fed 31 overweight and obese subjects:* Zhu L, Huang Y, Edirisinghe I, et al. "Using the Avocado to Test the Satiety Effects of a Fat-Fiber Combination in Place of Carbohydrate Energy in a Breakfast Meal in Overweight and Obese Men and Women: A Randomized Clinical Trial." *Nutrients.* 2019; 11(5): 952.

91 *"to discover and validate":* https://research.loveonetoday.com

91 *"avocados are a super food":* Hass Avocado Board. "Hass Avocado Board Reveals Major Avocado Nutrition Research Initiative." Press release. 2012; Mar. 12.

91 *trial sponsored by the Hass Avocado Board:* Henning SM, Yang J, Woo SL, et al. "Hass Avocado Inclusion in a Weight-Loss Diet Supported Weight Loss and Altered Gut Microbiota: A 12-Week Randomized, Parallel-Controlled Trial." *Current Developments in Nutrition.* 2019; 3(8): nzz068.

93 *spicy promises:* Shallow P. "Chili Peppers May Fire Up Weight Loss." CBSnews.com. 2015; Feb. 9; Garrard C. "13 Foods That Supercharge Your Metabolism." *Redbook.* 2017; Dec. 19; Stiehl C. "Is This the Number One Food for Weight Loss?" Eatthis.com. 2017; May 24.

93 *Danish study:* Westerterp-Plantenga MS, Smeets A, Lejeune MP. "Sensory and Gastrointestinal Satiety Effects of Capsaicin on Food Intake." *International Journal of Obesity.* 2005; 29(6): 682–8.

93 *Metabolism increased for several hours:* Ludy MJ, Mattes RD. "The Effects of Hedonically Acceptable Red Pepper Doses on Thermogenesis and Appetite." *Physiology & Behavior.* 2011; 102(3–4): 251–8.

93 *1-pound weight loss:* Ludy MJ, Moore GE, Mattes RD. "The Effects of Capsaicin and Capsiate on Energy Balance: Critical Review and Meta-Analyses of Studies in Humans." *Chemical Senses.* 2012; 37(2): 103–21.

94 *show larger upticks in calorie burning:* Zsiborás C, Mátics R, Hegyi P, et al. "Capsaicin and Capsiate Could Be Appropriate Agents for Treatment of Obesity: A Meta-Analysis of Human Studies." *Critical Reviews in Food Science and Nutrition.* 2018; 58(9): 1419–27.

94 *tracked people's weight:* Lejeune MP, Kovacs EM, Westerterp-Plantenga MS. "Effect of Capsaicin on Substrate Oxidation and Weight Maintenance after Modest Body-Weight Loss in Human Subjects." *British Journal of Nutrition.* 2003; 90(3): 651–9.

94-5 *one of the only published studies:* Hirsch AR, Gomez R. "Weight Reduction through Inhalation of Odorants." *Journal of Neurological and Orthopaedic Medicine and Surgery.* 1995; 16:28–31.

95 *scents may curb cravings:* Kemps E, Tiggemann M. "Olfactory Stimulation Curbs Food Cravings." *Addictive Behaviors.* 2013; 38(2): 1550–4.

95 *aromas can stimulate appetite:* Proserpio C, Invitti C, Boesveldt S, et al. "Ambient Odor Exposure Affects Food Intake and Sensory Specific Appetite in Obese Women." *Frontiers in Psychology.* 2019; 10: 7.

95 *observational studies:* Schwingshackl L, Hoffmann G, Kalle-Uhlmann T, et al. "Fruit and Vegetable Consumption and Changes in Anthropometric Variables in Adult Populations: A Systematic Review and Meta-Analysis of Prospective Cohort Studies." *PLOS One.* 2015; 10(10): e0140846.

95 *upping their intake of fruits, vegetables, and salads:* Han L, You D, Zeng F, et al. "Trends in Self-Perceived Weight Status, Weight Loss Attempts, and Weight Loss Strategies among Adults in the United States, 1999–2016." *JAMA Network Open.* 2019; 2(11): e1915219.

95 *among the most commonly reported weight-loss methods:* Martin CB, Herrick KA, Sarafrazi N, et al. "Attempts to Lose Weight among Adults in the United States, 2013–2016." *NCHS Data Brief.* 2018; (313).

95-6 *caveat isn't clear:* MacVean M. "Study: Fruits, Vegetables May Be Key to Long-Term Weight Loss." *Los Angeles Times.* 2012; Aug. 28; Barron B. "Rapid Weight Loss by Eating Fruits & Veggies." Livestrong.com. https://www.livestrong.com/article/46305-rapid-weight-loss-eating-fruits/

96 *Scottish study:* Whybrow S, Harrison CL, Mayer C, et al. "Effects of Added Fruits and Vegetables on Dietary Intakes and Body Weight in Scottish Adults." *British Journal of Nutrition.* 2006; 95(3): 496–503.

96 *review of this and other randomized trials:* Kaiser KA, Brown AW, Bohan Brown MM, et al. "Increased Fruit and Vegetable Intake Has No Discernible Effect on Weight Loss: A Systematic Review and Meta-Analysis." *American Journal of Clinical Nutrition.* 2014; 100(2): 567–76.

96 *Another such review:* Mytton OT, Nnoaham K, Eyles H, et al. "Systematic Review and Meta-Analysis of the Effect of Increased Vegetable and Fruit Consumption on Body Weight and Energy Intake." *BMC Public Health.* 2014; 14: 886.

97 *"To fight an epidemic of obesity":* University of Texas Health Science Center at Houston. "Farmer's Market Launched to Combat Obesity." *ScienceDaily.* 2009; Feb. 3.

97-8 *survey of 26 farmers' markets:* Lucan SC, Maroko AR, Sanon O, et al. "Urban Farmers' Markets: Accessibility, Offerings, and Produce Variety, Quality, and Price Compared to Nearby Stores." *Appetite.* 2015; 90: 23–30.

98 *results in better health:* de Oliveira Otto MC, Anderson CA, Dearborn JL, et al. "Dietary Diversity: Implications for Obesity Prevention in Adult Populations: A Science Advisory from the American Heart Association." *Circulation.* 2018; 138(11): e160–8.

98-9 *variety can prompt us to eat more:* Embling R, Pink AE, Gatzemeier J, et al. "Effect of Food Variety on Intake of a Meal: A Systematic Review and Meta-Analysis." *American Journal of Clinical Nutrition.* 2021; 113(3): 716–41.

99 *associated with better weight control:* Raynor HA, Jeffery RW, Phelan S, et al. "Amount of Food Group Variety Consumed in the Diet and Long-Term Weight Loss Maintenance." *Obesity Research.* 2005; 13(5): 883–90.

Chapter 5

103 *"the breakfast is the most important meal":* Cooper LS. "August Breakfasts." *Good Health.* 1917; 52(8): 389–90.

104 *"his innovative promotional techniques":* Carroll A. *Three Squares: The Invention of the American Meal.* New York: Basic Books. 2013; 146.

104 *1960s Grape-Nuts ad campaign:* https://www.youtube.com/watch?v=D8bNLOYgWO4

104-5 *published research supporting the claim:* Mattes RD. "Ready-to-Eat Cereal Used As a Meal Replacement Promotes Weight Loss in Humans." *Journal of the American College of Nutrition.* 2002; 21(6): 570–7; Shaw P, Walton J, Jakeman P. "The Effects of the Special K Challenge on Body Composition and Biomarkers of Metabolic Health in Healthy Adults." *Journal of Nutrition and Health Sciences.* 2015; 2(4): 403.

105 *influential study:* Cho S, Dietrich M, Brown CJ, et al. "The Effect of Breakfast Type on Total Daily Energy Intake and Body Mass Index: Results from the Third National Health and Nutrition Examination Survey (NHANES III)." *Journal of the American College of Nutrition.* 2003; 22(4): 296–302.

105 *Other observational studies:* Horikawa C, Kodama S, Yachi Y, et al. "Skipping Breakfast and Prevalence of Overweight and Obesity in Asian and Pacific Regions: A Meta-Analysis." *Preventive Medicine.* 2011; 53(4): 260–7.

105 *Pooling results from seven trials:* Sievert K, Hussain SM, Page MJ, et al. "Effect of Breakfast on Weight and Energy Intake: Systematic Review and Meta-Analysis of Randomised Controlled Trials." *BMJ.* 2019; 364: 142.

107 *six-week study:* Gillen JB, Percival ME, Ludzki A, et al. "Interval Training in the Fed or Fasted State Improves Body Composition and Muscle Oxidative Capacity in Overweight Women." *Obesity.* 2013; 21(11): 2249–55.

107 *review of this and other studies:* Hackett D, Hagstrom AD. "Effect of Overnight Fasted Exercise on Weight Loss and Body Composition: A Systematic Review and Meta-Analysis." *Journal of Functional Morphology and Kinesiology.* 2017; 2(4): 43.

107 *trumpeted in articles:* Drayer L. "When Trying to Lose Weight, Morning Meals Are Better Than Evening Ones." CNN.com. 2019; Oct. 14; Van Allen J. "Why Eating Late at Night May Be Particularly Bad for You and Your Diet." *Washington Post.* 2015; Aug. 24.

108 *study of Italians:* Bo S, Musso G, Beccuti G, et al. "Consuming More of Daily Caloric Intake at Dinner Predisposes to Obesity. A 6-Year Population-Based Prospective Cohort Study." *PLOS One.* 2014; 9(9): e108467.

108 *Israeli study:* Jakubowicz D, Barnea M, Wainstein J, et al. "High Caloric Intake at Breakfast vs. Dinner Differentially Influences Weight Loss of Overweight and Obese Women." *Obesity.* 2013; 21(12): 2504–12.

108 *no difference between smaller and larger dinners:* Fong M, Caterson ID, Madigan CD. "Are Large Dinners Associated with Excess Weight, and Does Eating a Smaller Dinner Achieve Greater Weight Loss? A Systematic Review and Meta-Analysis." *British Journal of Nutrition.* 2017; 118(8): 616–28.

108-9 *late chronotype:* Xiao Q, Garaulet M, Scheer FA. "Meal Timing and Obesity: Interactions with Macronutrient Intake and Chronotype." *International Journal of Obesity.* 2019; 43(9): 1701–11.

110 *food-combining diet produces no greater weight loss:* Golay A, Allaz AF, Ybarra J, et al. "Similar Weight Loss with Low-Energy Food Combining or Balanced Diets." *International Journal of Obesity.* 2000; 24(4): 492–6.

110 *subject of considerable research:* de Cabo R, Mattson MP. "Effects of Intermittent Fasting on Health, Aging, and Disease." *New England Journal of Medicine.* 2019; 381(26): 2541–51.

111 *researchers assigned 100 obese participants:* Trepanowski JF, Kroeger CM, Barnosky A, et al. "Effect of Alternate-Day Fasting on Weight Loss, Weight Maintenance, and Cardioprotection among Metabolically Healthy Obese Adults: A Randomized Clinical Trial." *JAMA Internal Medicine.* 2017; 177(7): 930–8.

111 *trial of more than 300 participants:* Headland ML, Clifton PM, Keogh JB. "Effect of Intermittent Compared to Continuous Energy Restriction on Weight Loss and Weight Maintenance after 12 Months in Healthy Overweight or Obese Adults." *International Journal of Obesity.* 2019; 43(10): 2028–36.

111 *smaller head-to-head comparisons:* Rynders CA, Thomas EA, Zaman A, et al. "Effectiveness of Intermittent Fasting and Time-Restricted Feeding Compared to Continuous Energy Restriction for Weight Loss." *Nutrients.* 2019; 11(10): 2442.

112 *dropout rates:* Welton S, Minty R, O'Driscoll T, et al. "Intermittent Fasting and Weight Loss: Systematic Review." *Canadian Family Physician.* 2020; 66(2): 117–25.

112 *greater loss of lean mass:* Lowe DA, Wu N, Rohdin-Bibby L, et al. "Effects of Time-Restricted Eating on Weight Loss and Other Metabolic Parameters in Women and Men with Overweight and Obesity: The TREAT Randomized Clinical Trial." *JAMA Internal Medicine.* 2020; 180(11): 1491–9.

114-5 *Europeans considered this practice uncivilized:* Carroll, op cit. 2.

115 *observational studies:* Canuto R, da Silva Garcez A, Kac G, et al. "Eating Frequency and Weight and Body Composition: A Systematic Review of Observational Studies." *Public Health Nutrition.* 2017; 20(12): 2079–95.

115 *researchers assigned 51 subjects:* Bachman JL, Raynor HA. "Effects of Manipulating Eating Frequency during a Behavioral Weight Loss Intervention: A Pilot Randomized Controlled Trial." *Obesity.* 2012; 20(5): 985–92.

115 *Virtually all other trials:* Kant AK. "Evidence for Efficacy and Effectiveness of Changes in Eating Frequency for Body Weight Management." *Advances in Nutrition.* 2014; 5(6): 822–8.

115 *grazing speeds metabolism is unproven:* La Bounty PM, Campbell BI, Wilson J, et al. "International Society of Sports Nutrition Position Stand: Meal Frequency." *Journal of the International Society of Sports Nutrition.* 2011; 8: 4.

117 *research doesn't provide clear answers:* Njike VY, Smith TM, Shuval O, et al. "Snack Food, Satiety, and Weight." *Advances in Nutrition.* 2016; 7(5): 866–78.

117 *"It's so simple":* quote from Krista Varady in Bakalar N. "Intermittent Fasting May Aid Weight Loss." *New York Times.* 2020; July 27.

Chapter 6

121 *research in the* Journal of the American Medical Association: Cutting WC, Mehrtens HG, Tainter ML. "Actions and Uses of Dinitrophenol: Promising Metabolic Applications." *Journal of the American Medical Association.* 1933; 101(3): 193–5.

122 *"toxic agent capable of inducing serious injury":* quoted in Colman E. "Dinitrophenol and Obesity: An Early Twentieth-Century Regulatory Dilemma." *Regulatory Toxicology and Pharmacology.* 2007; 48(2): 115–7.

122 *DNP-related deaths:* Sousa D, Carmo H, Bravo RR, et al. "Diet Aid or Aid to Die: An Update on 2, 4-Dinitrophenol (2, 4-DNP) Use as a Weight-Loss Product." *Archives of Toxicology.* 2020; 94(4): 1071–83.

122 *contain the prescription appetite suppressant sibutramine:* Tucker J, Fischer T, Upjohn L, et al. "Unapproved Pharmaceutical Ingredients Included in Dietary Supplements Associated with US Food and Drug Administration Warnings." *JAMA Network Open.* 2018; 1(6): e183337.

123 *ephedra and DMAA:* Ibid.; Eichner S, Maguire M, Shea LA, et al. "Banned and Discouraged-Use Ingredients Found in Weight Loss Supplements." *Journal of the American Pharmacists Association.* 2016; 56(5): 538–43.

123 *$6 billion annually:* "Global Weight Loss Supplements Industry." 2020; Sept. www.reportlinker.com/p05960487/Global-Weight-Loss-Supplements-Industry.html

123 *modestly boost metabolism and fat burning:* Jeukendrup AE, Randell R. "Fat Burners: Nutrition Supplements That Increase Fat Metabolism." *Obesity Reviews.* 2011; 12(10): 841–51.

123 *frequently cited study on caffeine and weight:* Lopez-Garcia E, van Dam RM, Rajpathak S, et al. "Changes in Caffeine Intake and Long-Term Weight Change in Men and Women." *American Journal of Clinical Nutrition.* 2006; 83(3): 674–80.

124 *combine caffeine with other substances:* For example, see Ohara T, Muroyama K, Yamamoto Y, et al. "Oral Intake of a Combination of Glucosyl Hesperidin and Caffeine Elicits an Anti-Obesity Effect in Healthy, Moderately Obese Subjects: A Randomized Double-Blind Placebo Controlled Trial." *Nutrition Journal.* 2016; 15: 6.

124 *claim that it can curb appetite:* Panek-Shirley LM, DeNysschen C, O'Brien E, et al. "Caffeine Transiently Affects Food Intake at Breakfast." *Journal of the Academy of Nutrition and Dietetics.* 2018; 118(10): 1832–43.

124 *study of adverse events reported to the FDA:* Jagim AR, Harty PS, Fischer KM, et al. "Adverse Events Reported to the United States Food and Drug Administration Related to Caffeine-Containing Products." *Mayo Clinic Proceedings.* 2020: 95(8): 1594–1603.

124 *combination of EGCG and caffeine:* Dulloo AG, Duret C, Rohrer D, et al. "Efficacy of a Green Tea Extract Rich in Catechin Polyphenols and Caffeine in Increasing 24-H Energy Expenditure and Fat Oxidation in Humans." *American Journal of Clinical Nutrition.* 1999; 70(6): 1040–5.

124 *pooled results from seven trials:* Maunder A, Bessell E, Lauche R, et al. "Effectiveness of Herbal Medicines for Weight Loss: A Systematic Review and Meta-Analysis of Randomized Controlled Trials." *Diabetes, Obesity and Metabolism.* 2020; 22(6): 891–903.

125 *"not likely . . . clinically important":* Jurgens TM, Whelan AM, Killian L, et al. "Green Tea for Weight Loss and Weight Maintenance in Overweight or Obese Adults." *Cochrane Database of Systematic Reviews.* 2012; 12.

125 *linked to liver damage:* Oketch-Rabah HA, Roe AL, Rider CV, et al. "United States Pharmacopeia (USP) Comprehensive Review of the Hepatotoxicity of Green Tea Extracts." *Toxicology Reports.* 2020; 7: 386–402.

125 *chlorogenic acid:* Tajik N, Tajik M, Mack I, et al. "The Potential Effects of Chlorogenic Acid, the Main Phenolic Components in Coffee, on Health: A Comprehensive Review of the Literature." *European Journal of Nutrition.* 2017; 56(7): 2215–44.

125 *review of 15 randomized trials:* Asbaghi O, Sadeghian M, Rahmani S, et al. "The Effect of Green Coffee Extract Supplementation on Anthropometric Measures in Adults: A Comprehensive Systematic Review and Dose-Response Meta-Analysis of Randomized Clinical Trials." *Complementary Therapies in Medicine.* 2020; 51: 102424.

125 *"green coffee extract is not recommended":* Buchanan R, Beckett RD. "Green Coffee for Pharmacological Weight Loss." *Journal of Evidence-Based Complementary & Alternative Medicine.* 2013; 18(4): 309–13.

126 *small effect on weight loss, which decreases over time:* Talenezhad N, Mohammadi M, Ramezani-Jolfaie N, et al. "Effects of L-Carnitine Supplementation on Weight Loss and Body Composition: A Systematic Review and Meta-Analysis of 37 Randomized Controlled Clinical Trials with Dose-Response Analysis." *Clinical Nutrition ESPEN.* 2020; 37: 9–23; Pooyandjoo M, Nouhi M, Shab-Bidar S, et al. "The Effect of (L-)Carnitine on Weight Loss in Adults: A Systematic Review and Meta-Analysis of Randomized Controlled Trials." *Obesity Reviews.* 2016; 17(10): 970–6.

126 *elevated risk of cardiovascular disease:* Koeth RA, Lam-Galvez BR, Kirsop J, et al. "L-Carnitine in Omnivorous Diets Induces an Atherogenic Gut Microbial Pathway in Humans." *Journal of Clinical Investigation.* 2019; 129(1): 373–87.

126 *leads to lower weight, but just barely:* Wharton S, Bonder R, Jeffery A, et al. "The Safety and Effectiveness of Commonly-Marketed Natural Supplements for Weight Loss in Populations with Obesity: A Critical Review of the Literature from 2006 to 2016." *Critical Reviews in Food Science and Nutrition.* 2020; 60(10): 1614–30.

126 *calls the evidence "insufficient":* Ibid.

126 *turned up no improvement:* Ibid.

126 *only a few trials, all of which are small:* Ríos-Hoyo A, Gutiérrez-Salmeán G. "New Dietary Supplements for Obesity: What We Currently Know." *Current Obesity Reports.* 2016; 5(2): 262–70.

126 *studies have found effects on weight:* Andueza N, Giner RM, Portillo MP. "Risks Associated with the Use of Garcinia as a Nutritional Complement to Lose Weight." *Nutrients.* 2021; 13(2): 450.

126 *linked to liver damage and psychiatric disorders:* Ibid.

126 *Overall, research is mixed:* Wharton, op cit.

126 *analysis pooling results from eight trials:* Onakpoya I, Posadzki P, Ernst E. "The Efficacy of Glucomannan Supplementation in Overweight and Obesity: A Systematic Review and Meta-Analysis of Randomized Clinical Trials." *Journal of the American College of Nutrition.* 2014; 33(1): 70–8.

127 *harmful effects on the heart:* Bredsdorff L, Wedebye EB, Nikolov NG, et al. "Raspberry Ketone in Food Supplements—High Intake, Few Toxicity Data—A Cause for Safety Concern?" *Regulatory Toxicology and Pharmacology.* 2015; 73(1): 196–200.

127 *interact with prescription medications:* Barrea L, Altieri B, Polese B, et al. "Nutritionist and Obesity: Brief Overview on Efficacy, Safety, and Drug Interactions of the Main Weight-Loss Dietary Supplements." *International Journal of Obesity Supplements.* 2019; 9(1): 32–49.

128 *eating more protein:* Wycherley TP, Moran LJ, Clifton PM, et al. "Effects of Energy-Restricted High-Protein, Low-Fat Compared with Standard-Protein, Low-Fat Diets: A Meta-Analysis of Randomized Controlled Trials." *American Journal of Clinical Nutrition.* 2012; 96(6): 1281–98.

128 *150 people who had lost weight:* Kjølbæk L, Sørensen LB, Søndertoft NB, et al. "Protein Supplements after Weight Loss Do Not Improve Weight Maintenance Compared with Recommended Dietary Protein Intake Despite Beneficial Effects on Appetite Sensation and Energy Expenditure: A Randomized, Controlled, Double-Blinded Trial." *American Journal of Clinical Nutrition.* 2017; 106(2): 684–97.

128 *article in* Good Housekeeping: Wiley HW, Pierce AL. "Swindled Getting Slim." *Good Housekeeping.* 1914; 58(1): 109–13.

129 *Such ads:* These descriptions came from ads in the 1910s for Kellogg's Safe Fat Reducer, Berdelet's Tablets, and Fell's Reducing Tablets.

130 *"Get high school skinny":* FTC. "FTC Approves Final Orders Banning Marketer behind 'Fat Burner' Diet Pills from Making or Selling Weight-Loss Products." 2014; Oct. 24. https://www.ftc.gov/news-events/press-releases/2014/10/ ftc-approves-final-orders-banning-marketer-behind-fat-burner-diet

130 *"You can keep eating":* FTC. "Portland, Maine Weight-Loss Supplement Sellers to Stop Deceptive Advertising, Illegal Billing Practices Following Joint FTC and Maine Attorney General Action." 2016; Feb. 5. https://www.ftc.gov/news-events/press-releases/2016/02/ portland-maine-weight-loss-supplement-sellers-stop-deceptive

130 *"Hi! CNN says this is one of the best.":* FTC. "FTC Charges Marketers Used Massive Spam Campaign to Pitch Bogus Weight-Loss Products." 2016; June 6. https://www.ftc.gov/news-events/press-releases/2016/06/ ftc-charges-marketers-used-massive-spam-campaign-pitch-bogus

131 *"Lost an average of 10%":* FTC. "Green Coffee Bean Manufacturer Settles FTC Charges of Pushing Its Product Based on Results of 'Seriously Flawed' Weight-Loss Study." 2014; Sept. 8. https://www.ftc.gov/news-events/press-releases/2014/09/ green-coffee-bean-manufacturer-settles-ftc-charges-pushing its

131 *research was published:* Vinson JA, Burnham BR, et al. "Randomized, Double-Blind, Placebo-Controlled, Linear Dose, Crossover Study to Evaluate the Efficacy and Safety of a Green Coffee Bean Extract in Overweight Subjects." *Diabetes, Metabolic Syndrome and Obesity: Targets and Therapy.* 2012; 5: 21–7.

135 *produced mixed results:* Brusaferro A, Cozzali R, Orabona C, et al. "Is It Time to Use Probiotics to Prevent or Treat Obesity?" *Nutrients.* 2018; 10(11): 1613; Borgeraas H, Johnson LK, Skattebu J, et al. "Effects of Probiotics on Body Weight, Body Mass Index, Fat Mass and Fat Percentage in Subjects with Overweight or Obesity: A Systematic Review and Meta-Analysis of Randomized Controlled Trials." *Obesity Reviews.* 2018; 19(2): 219–32.

135 *include plenty of fiber:* Myhrstad MC, Tunsjø H, Charnock C, et al. "Dietary Fiber, Gut Microbiota, and Metabolic Regulation—Current Status in Human Randomized Trials." *Nutrients.* 2020; 12(3): 859.

136 *1940s brought rainbow pills:* For an excellent history, see Cohen PA, Goday A, Swann JP. "The Return of Rainbow Diet Pills." *American Journal of Public Health.* 2012; 102(9): 1676–86.

136-7 *weight loss of more than 25 pounds:* Weintraub M, Sundaresan PR, Schuster B, et al. "Long-Term Weight Control Study II (Weeks 34 to 104) An Open-Label Study of Continuous Fenfluramine Plus Phentermine versus Targeted Intermittent Medication as Adjuncts to Behavior Modification, Caloric Restriction, and Exercise." *Clinical Pharmacology & Therapeutics.* 1992; 51(5): 595–601.

137 *told the* Wall Street Journal: Langreth R. "Critics Claim Drugs Intended for Obesity Are Often Misused." *Wall Street Journal.* 1997; Mar. 31.

137 *most important weight-loss discovery:* Levine S. *The Redux Revolution: Everything You Need to Know about the Most Important Weight-Loss Discovery of the Century.* William Morrow. 1996.

137 *doctors at the Mayo Clinic:* Connolly HM, Crary JL, McGoon MD, et al. "Valvular Heart Disease Associated with Fenfluramine-Phentermine." *New England Journal of Medicine.* 1997; 337(9): 581–8.

138 *shave off roughly 5 to 20 more pounds:* Khera R, Murad MH, Chandar AK, et al. "Association of Pharmacological Treatments for Obesity with Weight Loss and Adverse Events: A Systematic Review and Meta-Analysis." *JAMA.* 2016; 315(22): 2424–34.

138 *lose at least 5 percent of their weight:* LeBlanc ES, Patnode CD, Webber EM, et al. "Behavioral and Pharmacotherapy Weight Loss Interventions to Prevent Obesity-Related Morbidity and Mortality in Adults: Updated Evidence Report and Systematic Review for the US Preventive Services Task Force." *JAMA.* 2018; 320(11): 1172–91.

139 *dropout rates of up to 45 percent:* Khera, op cit.

139 *By one estimate:* Elangovan A, Shah R, Smith ZL. "Pharmacotherapy for Obesity—Trends Using a Population Level National Database." *Obesity Surgery.* 2021; 31(3): 1105–12.

140 *Estrogen replacement therapy:* National Cancer Institute. "Menopausal Hormone Therapy and Cancer." https://www.cancer.gov/about-cancer/ causes-prevention/risk/hormones/mht-fact-sheet

140 *testosterone therapy:* Gagliano-Jucá T, Basaria S. "Testosterone Replacement Therapy and Cardiovascular Risk." *Nature Reviews Cardiology.* 2019; 16(9): 555–74.

140 *"bioidentical" hormones:* National Academies of Sciences, Engineering, and Medicine. *The Clinical Utility of Compounded Bioidentical Hormone Therapy: A Review of Safety, Effectiveness, and Use.* Washington, DC: National Academies Press. 2020.

140 *congressional hearing:* US Senate Committee on Commerce, Science, and Transportation. "Protecting Consumers from False and Deceptive Advertising of Weight-Loss Products." 2014; June 17. https://www.commerce.senate. gov/2014/6/commerce-committee-announces-subcommittee-hearing-on-false-and-deceptive-marketing-of-weight-loss-products

141 *study of visits to hospital emergency departments:* Geller AI, Shehab N, Weidle NJ, et al. "Emergency Department Visits for Adverse Events Related to Dietary Supplements." *New England Journal of Medicine.* 2015; 373(16): 1531–40.

141 *flawed and woefully underutilized:* For details, see Starr RR. "Too Little, Too Late: Ineffective Regulation of Dietary Supplements in the United States." *American Journal of Public Health.* 2015; 105(3): 478–85.

141 *study involving women who wanted to lose weight:* Chang YY, Chiou WB. "The Liberating Effect of Weight Loss Supplements on Dietary Control: A Field Experiment." *Nutrition.* 2014; 30(9): 1007–10.

Chapter 7

145 *collection of penny scales:* www.theamericanweigh.com

147 *policyholders past their early to mid-30s:* Weigley ES. "Average? Ideal? Desirable? A Brief Overview of Height-Weight Tables in the United States." *Journal of the American Dietetic Association.* 1984; 84(4): 417–23.

148 *1972 study:* Keys A, Fidanza F, Karvonen MJ, et al. "Indices of Relative Weight and Obesity." *Journal of Chronic Diseases.* 1972; 25(6–7): 329–43.

148 *"a simple measurement":* "National Implications of Obesity." NIH Consensus Statement. 1985; 5(9): 1–7.

149 *BMI misses half:* Okorodudu DO, Jumean MF, Montori VM, et al. "Diagnostic Performance of Body Mass Index to Identify Obesity as Defined by Body Adiposity: A Systematic Review and Meta-Analysis." *International Journal of Obesity.* 2010; 34(5): 791–9.

150 *have heavier bones:* Wagner DR, Heyward VH. "Measures of Body Composition in Blacks and Whites: A Comparative Review." *American Journal of Clinical Nutrition.* 2000; 71(6): 1392–402.

150 *cause BMI to underestimate:* Deurenberg P, Deurenberg-Yap M, Guricci S. "Asians Are Different from Caucasians and from Each Other in Their Body Mass Index/Body Fat Per Cent Relationship." *Obesity Reviews.* 2002; 3(3): 141–6.

150 *greater risk of heart disease:* Piché ME, Poirier P, Lemieux I, et al. "Overview of Epidemiology and Contribution of Obesity and Body Fat Distribution to Cardiovascular Disease: An Update." *Progress in Cardiovascular Diseases.* 2018; 61(2): 103–13.

150 *more than 40,000 adults:* Tomiyama AJ, Hunger JM, Nguyen-Cuu J, et al. "Misclassification of Cardiometabolic Health When Using Body Mass Index Categories in NHANES 2005–2012." *International Journal of Obesity.* 2016; 40(5): 883–6.

151 *research that has followed:* Caleyachetty R, Thomas GN, Toulis KA, et al. "Metabolically Healthy Obese and Incident Cardiovascular Disease Events among 3.5 Million Men and Women." *Journal of the American College of Cardiology.* 2017; 70(12): 1429–37; Bell JA, Kivimaki M, Hamer M. "Metabolically Healthy Obesity and Risk of Incident Type 2 Diabetes: A Meta-Analysis of Prospective Cohort Studies." *Obesity Reviews.* 2014; 15(6): 504–15.

151 *greater risk of premature death:* Cerhan JR, Moore SC, Jacobs EJ, et al. "A Pooled Analysis of Waist Circumference and Mortality in 650,000 Adults." *Mayo Clinic Proceedings.* 2014; 89(3): 335–45.

151 *thresholds aren't optimal:* Ross R, Neeland IJ, Yamashita S, et al. "Waist Circumference As a Vital Sign in Clinical Practice: A Consensus Statement from the IAS and ICCR Working Group on Visceral Obesity." *Nature Reviews Endocrinology.* 2020; 16(3): 177–89.

152 *"Despite all the progress":* Karasu SR. "Adolphe Quetelet and the Evolution of Body Mass Index (BMI)." Psychologytoday.com. 2016; Mar. 18.

152 *test of six home scales:* Byrne S. "Body-Fat Scale Review." Consumerreports.org. 2016; Mar. 11.

153-4 *"made women feel humiliated":* Fraser L. *Losing It: America's Obsession with Weight and the Industry That Feeds on It.* New York: Dutton. 1997; 38.

154 *1932 article:* Boyd A. "How the Stars Stay Slim and Trim." *New Movie Magazine.* 1932; Jan.: 80.

154 *BMIs steadily declined:* Byrd-Bredbenner C, Murray J, Schlussel YR. "Temporal Changes in Anthropometric Measurements of Idealized Females and Young Women in General." *Women & Health.* 2005; 41(2): 13–30.

154 *falling into the "underweight" category:* Rubinstein S, Caballero B. "Is Miss America an Undernourished Role Model?" *JAMA.* 2000; 283(12): 1569.

155 *"conspicuously thin":* Conlin L, Bissell K. "Beauty Ideals in the Checkout Aisle: Health-Related Messages in Women's Fashion and Fitness Magazines." *Journal of Magazine & New Media Research.* 2014; 15(2): 1–19.

155 *100 most-followed females:* Ho C. "Decoding the Instagram Beauty Standard." YouTube. 2019; Sept. 16. www.youtube.com/watch?v=5HJ8du5i_rE

155 *internalize the thin body ideal:* Mingoia J, Hutchinson AD, Wilson C, et al. "The Relationship between Social Networking Site Use and the Internalization of a Thin Ideal in Females: A Meta-Analytic Review." *Frontiers in Psychology.* 2017; 8: 1351.

155 *middle-aged and older women:* Cameron E, Ward P, Mandville-Anstey SA, et al. "The Female Aging Body: A Systematic Review of Female Perspectives on Aging, Health, and Body Image." *Journal of Women & Aging.* 2019; 31(1): 3–17; McCabe MP, Ricciardelli LA, James T. "A Longitudinal Study of Body Change Strategies of Fitness Center Attendees." *Eating Behaviors.* 2007; 8(4): 492–6.

155 *In men:* Blond A. "Impacts of Exposure to Images of Ideal Bodies on Male Body Dissatisfaction: A Review." *Body Image.* 2008; 5(3): 244–50.

157 *study of 12,000 people:* Christakis NA, Fowler JH. "The Spread of Obesity in a Large Social Network over 32 Years." *New England Journal of Medicine.* 2007; 357(4): 370–9.

157 *research involving military families:* Datar A, Nicosia N. "Assessing Social Contagion in Body Mass Index, Overweight, and Obesity Using a Natural Experiment." *JAMA Pediatrics.* 2018; 172(3): 239–46.

157 *more likely to lose weight:* Gorin AA, Lenz EM, Cornelius T, et al. "Randomized Controlled Trial Examining the Ripple Effect of a Nationally Available Weight Management Program on Untreated Spouses." *Obesity.* 2018; 26(3): 499–504; Leahey TM, LaRose JG, Fava JL, et al. "Social Influences Are Associated with BMI and Weight Loss Intentions in Young Adults." *Obesity.* 2011; 19(6): 1157–62.

158 *widely cited study:* Foster GD, Wadden TA, Vogt RA, et al. "What Is a Reasonable Weight Loss? Patients' Expectations and Evaluations of Obesity Treatment Outcomes." *Journal of Consulting and Clinical Psychology.* 1997; 65(1): 79–85.

158 *tend to be unrealistic:* Pétré B, Scheen A, Ziegler O, et al. "Weight Loss Expectations and Determinants in a Large Community-Based Sample." *Preventive Medicine Reports.* 2018; 12:12–9; Dalle Grave R, Calugi S, Compare A, et al. "Weight Loss Expectations and Attrition in Treatment-Seeking Obese Women." *Obesity Facts.* 2015; 8(5): 311–8.

158 *expectations tend to be highest:* Wamsteker EW, Geenen R, Zelissen PM, et al. "Unrealistic Weight-Loss Goals among Obese Patients Are Associated with Age and Causal Attributions." *Journal of the American Dietetic Association.* 2009; 109(11): 1903–8; Fabricatore AN, Wadden TA, Rohay JM, et al. "Weight Loss Expectations and Goals in a Population Sample of Overweight and Obese US Adults." *Obesity.* 2008; 16(11): 2445–50.

158-9 *survey of primary care physicians:* Phelan S, Nallari M, Darroch FE, et al. "What Do Physicians Recommend to Their Overweight and Obese Patients?" *Journal of the American Board of Family Medicine.* 2009; 22(2): 115–22.

159 *linked to health benefits:* Ryan DH, Yockey SR. "Weight Loss and Improvement in Comorbidity: Differences at 5%, 10%, 15%, and Over." *Current Obesity Reports.* 2017; 6(2): 187–94.

159 *Italian study of nearly 1,800 people:* Dalle Grave R, Calugi S, Molinari E, et al. "Weight Loss Expectations in Obese Patients and Treatment Attrition: An Observational Multicenter Study." *Obesity Research.* 2005; 13(11): 1961–9.

159 *not all studies show:* Crawford R, Glover L. "The Impact of Pre-Treatment Weight-Loss Expectations on Weight Loss, Weight Regain, and Attrition in People Who Are Overweight and Obese: A Systematic Review of the Literature." *British Journal of Health Psychology.* 2012; 17(3): 609–30.

159-60 *study of middle-aged people:* Olson EA, Visek AJ, McDonnell KA, et al. "Thinness Expectations and Weight Cycling in a Sample of Middle-Aged Adults." *Eating Behaviors.* 2012; 13(2): 142–5.

160 *research overall is inconclusive:* Mehta T, Smith DL, Muhammad J, et al. "Impact of Weight Cycling on Risk of Morbidity and Mortality." *Obesity Reviews.* 2014; 15(11): 870–81.

160 *greater fat accumulation and an increased risk of diabetes:* Cereda E, Malavazos AE, Caccialanza R, et al. "Weight Cycling Is Associated with Body Weight Excess and Abdominal Fat Accumulation: A Cross-Sectional Study." *Clinical Nutrition.* 2011; 30(6): 718–23; Zou H, Yin P, Liu L, et al. "Association between Weight Cycling and Risk of Developing Diabetes in Adults: A Systematic Review and Meta-Analysis." *Journal of Diabetes Investigation.* 2021; 12(4): 625–32.

160-1 *"Unless you want to battle evolution":* Mann T. *Secrets from the Eating Lab: The Science of Weight Loss, the Myth of Willpower, and Why You Should Never Diet Again.* New York: HarperWave. 2015; 31.

161 *review of 19 trials:* Shieh C, Knisely MR, Clark D, et al. "Self-Weighing in Weight Management Interventions: A Systematic Review of Literature." *Obesity Research & Clinical Practice.* 2016; 10(5): 493–519.

161 *negative psychological effects:* Benn Y, Webb TL, Chang BP, et al. "What Is the Psychological Impact of Self-Weighing? A Meta-Analysis." *Health Psychology Review.* 2016; 10(2): 187–203; Pacanowski CR, Linde JA, Neumark-Sztainer D. "Self-Weighing: Helpful or Harmful for Psychological Well-Being? A Review of the Literature." *Current Obesity Reports.* 2015; 4(1): 65–72.

162 *experience a number of benefits:* Ryan, op cit.

162-3 *"Loving yourself":* deVos K. "The Problem with Body Positivity." *New York Times.* 2018; May 29.

163 *"while living the healthiest lifestyle":* Freedhoff Y, Sharma AM. *Best Weight: A Practical Guide to Office-Based Obesity Management.* Canadian Obesity Network. 2010; 12.

Chapter 8

165 *secrets:* "Best Diet Secrets." *Health.* 2014; Oct.; "One-Minute Summer Weight Loss Secrets." *Prevention.* 2018; June; "Weight Loss Secrets Only Nutritionists Know." *Women's Health.* 2016; Aug. 15; "20+ More Stars' Secrets Inside." *Us Weekly.* 2021; Jan. 11.

165 *shortcut:* "13 Shortcuts to Lasting Weight Loss." *Redbook.* 2017; Feb.; "7 Weight Loss Shortcuts That Actually Work." *Women's Health.* 2015; Jan. 9.; "#1 Weight Loss Shortcut." *Women's World.* 2021; Jan. 18.

165 *14 popular diet plans:* Hitchcock C, Svendrovski A, Kiflen R, et al. "Comparison of Dietary Macronutrient Patterns Based on 14 Popular Named Dietary Programs for Weight and Cardiovascular Risk Reduction in Adults: A Systematic Review and Network Meta-Analysis of Randomized Trials." *BMJ.* 2020; 369: m696.

166 *"plethora of choice":* Truby H, Haines TP. "Comparative Weight Loss with Popular Diets." *BMJ.* 2020; 369: m1269.

166 *"finding a set of behaviors":* Catenacci VA, Odgen L, Phelan S, et al. "Dietary Habits and Weight Maintenance Success in High Versus Low Exercisers in the National Weight Control Registry." *Journal of Physical Activity and Health.* 2014; 11(8): 1540–8.

167 *eat roughly the same volume:* Bell EA, Castellanos VH, Pelkman CL, et al. "Energy Density of Foods Affects Energy Intake in Normal-Weight Women." *American Journal of Clinical Nutrition.* 1998; 67(3): 412–20.

167 *sneaked pureed vegetables into entrées:* Blatt AD, Roe LS, Rolls BJ. "Hidden Vegetables: An Effective Strategy to Reduce Energy Intake and Increase Vegetable Intake in Adults." *American Journal of Clinical Nutrition.* 2011; 93(4): 756–63.

167 *trial involving 132 overweight subjects:* Lowe MR, Butryn ML, Thomas JG, et al. "Meal Replacements, Reduced Energy Density Eating, and Weight Loss Maintenance in Primary Care Patients: A Randomized Controlled Trial." *Obesity.* 2014; 22(1): 94–100.

167 *study that tracked women for six years:* Savage JS, Marini M, Birch LL. "Dietary Energy Density Predicts Women's Weight Change over 6 Years." *American Journal of Clinical Nutrition.* 2008; 88(3): 677–84.

168 *research is mixed:* Kjølbæk L, Sørensen LB, Søndertoft NB, et al. "Protein Supplements after Weight Loss Do Not Improve Weight Maintenance Compared with Recommended Dietary Protein Intake Despite Beneficial Effects on Appetite Sensation and Energy Expenditure: A Randomized, Controlled, Double-Blinded Trial." *American Journal of Clinical Nutrition.* 2017; 106(2): 684–97; Westerterp-Plantenga MS, Lemmens SG, Westerterp KR. "Dietary Protein—Its Role in Satiety, Energetics, Weight Loss and Health." *British Journal of Nutrition.* 2012; 108(S2): S105–12.

168 *drinking your calories:* Pan A, Hu FB. "Effects of Carbohydrates on Satiety: Differences between Liquid and Solid Food." *Current Opinion in Clinical Nutrition and Metabolic Care.* 2011; 14(4): 385–90.

169 *weight-control registries in five countries:* Paixão C, Dias CM, Jorge R, et al. "Successful Weight Loss Maintenance: A Systematic Review of Weight Control Registries." *Obesity Reviews.* 2020; 21(5): e13003.

171 *linked insufficient sleep to obesity:* Wu Y, Zhai L, Zhang D. "Sleep Duration and Obesity among Adults: A Meta-Analysis of Prospective Studies." *Sleep Medicine.* 2014; 15(12): 1456–62.

171 *study that followed more than 68,000 women:* Patel SR, Malhotra A, White DP, et al. "Association between Reduced Sleep and Weight Gain in Women." *American Journal of Epidemiology.* 2006; 164(10): 947–54.

171 *assigned 200 subjects to sleep for only four hours:* Spaeth AM, Dinges DF, Goel N. "Effects of Experimental Sleep Restriction on Weight Gain, Caloric Intake, and Meal Timing in Healthy Adults." *Sleep.* 2013; 36(7): 981–90.

171 *results from this trial and 10 others:* Al Khatib HK, Harding SV, Darzi J, et al. "The Effects of Partial Sleep Deprivation on Energy Balance: A Systematic Review and Meta-Analysis." *European Journal of Clinical Nutrition.* 2017; 71(5): 614–24.

171 *not all, support this idea:* Zhu B, Shi C, Park CG, et al. "Effects of Sleep Restriction on Metabolism-Related Parameters in Healthy Adults: A Comprehensive Review and Meta-Analysis of Randomized Controlled Trials." *Sleep Medicine Reviews.* 2019; 45: 18–30.

171 *make the body less sensitive to insulin:* Ibid.

171 *associated with a number of conditions:* Itani O, Jike M, Watanabe N, et al. "Short Sleep Duration and Health Outcomes: A Systematic Review, Meta-Analysis, and Meta-Regression." *Sleep Medicine.* 2017; 32: 246–56; Patyar S, Patyar RR. "Correlation between Sleep Duration and Risk of Stroke." *Journal of Stroke and Cerebrovascular Diseases.* 2015; 24(5): 905–11; Zhai L, Zhang H, Zhang D. "Sleep Duration and Depression among Adults: A Meta-Analysis of Prospective Studies." *Depression & Anxiety.* 2015; 32(9): 664–70.

172 *study involving more than 2,500 people:* Jackson SE, Kirschbaum C, Steptoe A. "Hair Cortisol and Adiposity in a Population-Based Sample of 2,527 Men and Women Aged 54 to 87 Years." *Obesity.* 2017; 25(3): 539–44.

172 *American Psychological Association survey: Stress in America: Are Teens Adopting Adults' Stress Habits?* American Psychological Association. 2014; Feb. 11. https://www.apa.org/news/press/releases/stress/2013/stress-report.pdf

174 *study of successful losers in the NWCR:* Butryn ML, Phelan S, Hill JO, et al. "Consistent Self-Monitoring of Weight: A Key Component of Successful Weight Loss Maintenance." *Obesity.* 2007; 15(12): 3091–6.

175 *both short-term and long-term weight loss:* Burke LE, Wang J, Sevick MA. "Self-Monitoring in Weight Loss: A Systematic Review of the Literature." *Journal of the American Dietetic Association.* 2011; 111(1): 92–102; Laitner MH, Minski SA, Perri MG. "The Role of Self-Monitoring in the Maintenance of Weight Loss Success." *Eating Behaviors.* 2016; 21: 193–7.

175 *people who are the most diligent:* Harvey J, Krukowski R, Priest J, et al. "Log Often, Lose More: Electronic Dietary Self-Monitoring for Weight Loss." *Obesity.* 2019; 27(3): 380–4.

176 *study that surveyed food journalers:* Cordeiro F, Epstein DA, Thomaz E, et al. "Barriers and Negative Nudges: Exploring Challenges in Food Journaling." *Proceedings of the SIGCHI Conference on Human Factors in Computing Systems.* 2015; Apr.: 1159–62.

178 *implementation intentions can keep us from veering off course:* Gollwitzer PM, Sheeran P. "Implementation Intentions and Goal Achievement: A Meta-Analysis of Effects and Processes." *Advances in Experimental Social Psychology.* 2006; 38: 69–119.

180 *researchers surveyed nearly 5,000 members of WW:* Phelan S, Halfman T, Pinto AM, et al. "Behavioral and Psychological Strategies of Long-Term Weight Loss Maintainers in a Widely Available Weight Management Program." *Obesity.* 2020; 28(2): 421–8.

180 *"there will be ups and downs":* Suzanne Phelan, quoted in Brody JE. "How to Lose Weight and Keep It Off." *New York Times.* 2020; Mar. 16.

181 *nearly 90 trials involving behavioral therapy:* US Preventive Services Task Force. "Behavioral Weight Loss Interventions to Prevent Obesity-Related Morbidity and Mortality in Adults: US Preventive Services Task Force Recommendation Statement." *JAMA.* 2018; 320(11): 1163–71.

182 *study that included more than 1,100 subjects:* Adams TD, Davidson LE, Litwin SE, et al. "Weight and Metabolic Outcomes 12 Years after Gastric Bypass." *New England Journal of Medicine.* 2017; 377: 1143–55.

182 *surgery also improves:* Arterburn DE, Telem DA, Kushner RF, et al. "Benefits and Risks of Bariatric Surgery in Adults: A Review." *JAMA.* 2020; 324(9): 879–87; Carlsson LM, Sjöholm K, Jacobson P, et al. "Life Expectancy after Bariatric Surgery in the Swedish Obese Subjects Study." *New England Journal of Medicine.* 2020; 383(16): 1535–43.

INDEX

138
Cooper, Lenna Frances, 103
cortisol, 172

D

deVos, Kelly, 162–163
Diet and Health (Peters), 42
dietary fat
    calories per gram, 44
    low-fat diets, 24–28
    as weight-gain cause, 18–20
    as weight-loss aid, 88–92
dietary patterns. See food choices
Dietary Supplement Health and Education Act (DSHEA), 129, 140–141
Diet Cults (Fitzgerald), 22
DIETFITS study, 25
diet pills, 135–139, 142–143. See also weight-loss supplements
diets and dieting
    adherence to, 26–27
    Atkins diet, 20–22, 26
    banned foods in, 27–28, 38
    case study, 28–29
    comparison studies, 165–166
    DuPont diet, 21
    grapefruit diet, 84
    guidelines for, 38–39
    keto diet, 26, 27, 28–29
    low-fat versus low-carb, 24–26
    Ornish diet, 20, 26
    Twinkie Diet, 41–42
    werewolf (lunar) diet, 101
    yo-yo dieting, 57–58, 78, 159–160
diet soda, 55–56
digestion, 45–46
dinnertime, 107–109
DMAA, 123
DNP (2,4-dinitrophenol), 121–122
Dr. Atkins Diet Revolution (Atkins),

21–22
Drinking Man's Diet, The (Cameron), 21
DSHEA (Dietary Supplement Health and Education Act), 129, 140–141
DuPont diet, 21

E

eating disorders
    anorexia, 92
    binge eating, 27, 173
    fasting and, 112
    menu labeling and, 57
    unrealistic ideal weight and, 159
eat less, move more (ELMM), 64
EGCG (epigallocatechin gallate), 124
18-Day Diet, 84
ELMM (eat less, move more), 64
energy density of food, 167
ephedra, 123
epigallocatechin gallate (EGCG), 124
EPOC (excess postexercise oxygen consumption), 69
estrogen replacement therapy, 140
evening meals, 107–109
excess postexercise oxygen consumption (EPOC), 69
exercise
    aerobic, 76, 169
    amount recommended, 68, 75
    barriers to and motivation, 170
    calories expended by, 67–70
    case study, 78–79
    compensatory responses to, 70–73
    expectations and focus of, 79–82
    guidelines for, 82
    health benefits of, 76–78, 79
    in healthy lifestyle, 169–170
    intensity level of, 69–70
    resistance training, 76, 169–170

M

N

O

CPSIA information can be obtained
at www.ICGtesting.com
Printed in the USA
LVHW031545271021
701710LV00002B/297